UGOH ONYEMAIZU

65 ESSENTIAL SIMPLE EXERCISES FOR EVERY STAGE OF LIFE

STRENGTH AND VITALITY ASSURED

First edition

Contents

1

INTRODUCTION

It is possible that you would have searched the book shelves for manuscripts containing easy, simple, essential but useful contents for your daily exercise routines without any success. Welcome then to "65 Essential Simple Exercises for Every Stage of Life - Strength and Vitality Assured"! In this book, we'll explore the incredible benefits of regular exercises and how it can transform your body and your life. Whether you're a young adult, an adult, or a senior, the key to unlocking lasting vitality lies in incorporating simple, but yet effective exercises into your daily routine.

Throughout these pages, you'll discover a diverse range of exercises designed to target every major muscle group, improve flexibility, and boost overall vitality. From basic squats and lunges to gentle stretches and balance exercises, each movement is carefully selected to meet you where you are and help you reach your fitness goals. Were you aware that simple breathing exercises if done properly have the capacity to do great things to your health and overall well being?

We want our readers to note that the secret to achieving a great vitality lies in consistency and commitment to regular exercise. By incorporating these simple but sure exercises into your daily routine, you'll not only strengthen your muscles and improve your flexibility but also enhance your energy levels, mood, and overall well-being.

So, are you ready to take the first step towards a healthier, happier you? Let's drive in and discover the power of regular simple exercises in achieving lifelong strength and vitality!

2

BODYWEIGHT SQUATS EXERCISE

1. Bodyweight Squats:

Squat exercises don't always involve heavy barbells on your back. A simpler version of the squat exercise utilizes only your bodyweight.

Bodyweight squats engage your hip and glute muscles, strengthening these key areas without the need for additional weight. The glute muscles, located in the buttocks, are particularly targeted with each repetition. Additionally, secondary muscles such as the obliques, calves, and hamstrings also benefit from this exercise.

How to Perform Bodyweight Squats:

- Begin by standing straight with your feet hip-width apart.
- Slowly lower yourself by bending your knees, ensuring they remain directly over your toes without extending past them.
- Maintain focus on keeping your weight centered on your heels as you push yourself back up to a standing position.
- Concentrate on activating your hamstrings and glutes, emphasizing

the squeeze in your glute muscles as you rise. Repeat for additional repetitions.

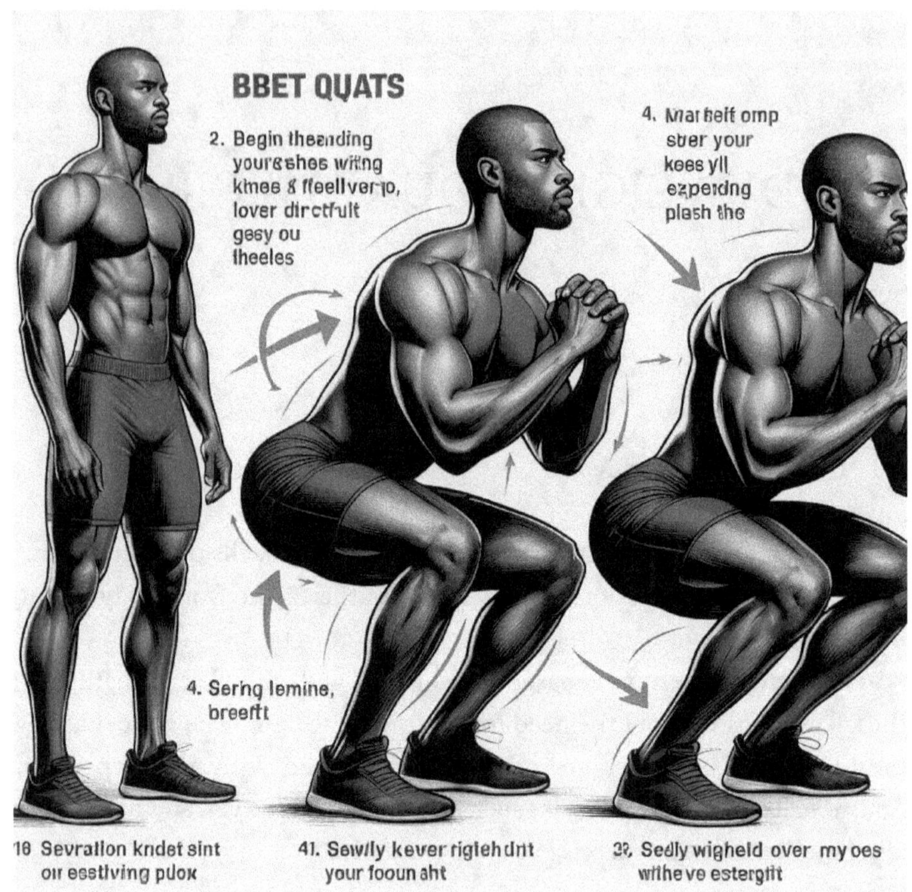

Benefits of Bodyweight Squats:

1. Strengthens Lower Body Muscles: Bodyweight squats primarily target the muscles of the lower body, including the quadriceps, hamstrings, and glutes. Regularly performing squats can help increase strength and endurance in these muscles.

2. Improves Functional Movement: Squatting is a functional movement

pattern that mimics everyday activities like sitting, standing, and bending down. By practicing bodyweight squats, you can improve your ability to perform these movements with ease and efficiency.

3. Enhances Core Stability: While performing bodyweight squats, your core muscles, including the abdominals and obliques, engage to stabilize your torso. This exercise is found to help improve overall core strength and stability.

4. Requires No Equipment: Bodyweight squats can be done anywhere and any time since they don't require any equipment. This makes them a convenient exercise option for those who may not have access to a gym or equipment.

5. Promotes Joint Health: Squatting through a full range of motion helps improve joint flexibility and mobility, particularly in the hips, knees, and ankles. This can contribute to better overall joint health and reduce the risk of injury.

6. Burns Calories: Squats are usually a compound exercise, which means that they engage multiple muscle groups simultaneously. As a result, they can help increase calorie expenditure and contribute to weight loss or weight management goals.

7. Improves Balance and Coordination: Squats challenge your balance and coordination, especially when performed with proper form. Over time, practicing bodyweight squats can help improve balance and coordination, which is essential for everyday activities and athletic performance.

8. Boosts Athletic Performance: Strong lower body muscles and improved functional movement patterns gained from bodyweight squats can translate to better performance in various sports and physical activities.

Incorporating bodyweight squats into your workout routine can offer a wide range of benefits for overall health, fitness, and performance.

NORMAL PLANK EXERCISE

2) Plank Exercise

The plank exercise stands as a cornerstone of isometric training, offering a multitude of benefits by engaging various muscle groups simultaneously. This static exercise targets the core muscles, including the abdominals, obliques, and lower back, while also recruiting muscles in the shoulders, arms, glutes, and legs for stabilization.

By assuming a plank position, you support your body weight on your forearms and toes, creating a straight line from head to heels. This posture challenges your core muscles to maintain stability and balance, while also activating the muscles in your arms, shoulders, and legs to keep your body aligned.

Performing the plank with proper form is essential to maximize its benefits and minimize the risk of injury.

How to Perform Plank Exercise:

- Begin in a kneeling position with your forearms resting flat on the ground, shoulder-width apart.

- Lift your body off the ground, extending your legs behind you and supporting your weight on your forearms and toes.
- Maintain a straight line from head to heels, engaging your core muscles to prevent sagging or arching in the lower back.
- Keep your shoulders stacked directly above your elbows, and your gaze focused slightly ahead of you to maintain proper alignment.
- Hold the plank position for the desired duration, focusing on steady breathing and engaging the core muscles throughout.

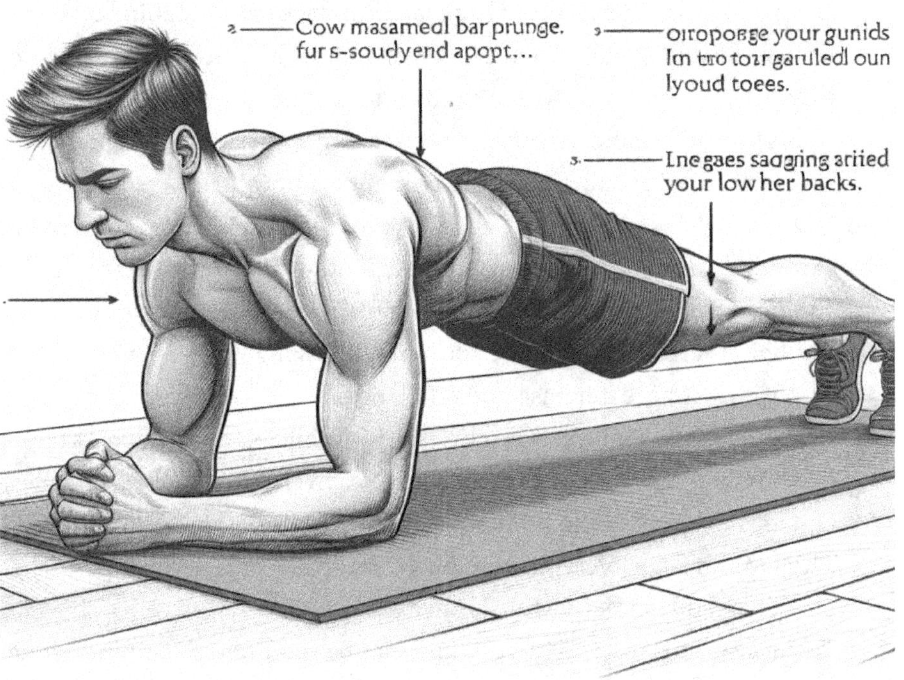

Benefits of Plank Exercise:

1. Core Strength: Planks primarily target the core muscles, including the rectus abdominis, transverse abdominis, obliques, and erector spinae. By engaging these muscles to maintain a stable position, planks effectively strengthen the entire core, which is essential for posture, balance, and spinal alignment.

2. Improved Posture: Strengthening the core muscles through plank exercises can help improve overall posture by promoting better spinal alignment and reducing the risk of slouching or rounding of the shoulders.

3. Reduced Risk of Back Pain: Strong core muscles play a crucial role in supporting the spine and reducing the risk of back pain or injury. Planks target the deep stabilizing muscles of the core, which can help alleviate strain on the lower back and improve spinal stability.

4. Enhanced Stability and Balance: Planks require activation of the muscles throughout the body to maintain a stable position. By improving stability and balance, plank exercises can enhance performance in various activities and reduce the risk of falls or injuries.

5. Increased Muscular Endurance: Holding a plank position for an extended period challenges muscular endurance, particularly in the core muscles. Regularly incorporating plank exercises into your routine can help increase muscular endurance, allowing you to perform daily activities with greater ease and efficiency.

6. Engagement of Multiple Muscle Groups: While planks primarily target the core muscles, they also engage muscles in the shoulders, arms, chest, and legs to support the body's weight and maintain proper alignment. This comprehensive engagement of multiple muscle groups makes planks a highly effective full-body exercise.

7. Versatility and Accessibility: Planks can be modified to suit individual fitness levels and goals, making them accessible to people of all fitness levels. Whether performed on the forearms or hands, with extended or bent knees, planks can be tailored to accommodate different abilities

and preferences.

8. Improved Athletic Performance: Strong core muscles are essential for optimal athletic performance in various sports and activities. By strengthening the core and enhancing overall stability and balance, plank exercises can improve athletic performance and reduce the risk of sports-related injuries.

When plank exercises are regularly incorporated into your fitness routine, it can offer a wide range of benefits for core strength, stability, posture, and overall physical health. Whether you're a beginner or an experienced athlete, planks can be an effective addition to your workout regimen.

4

PUSH-UP EXERCISE

3) Push-Up Exercise

Push-ups are a classic bodyweight exercise renowned for their effectiveness in targeting multiple muscle groups simultaneously. This compound exercise not only builds strength and endurance but also enhances muscular definition, making it a staple in fitness routines worldwide.

Push-ups primarily target the upper body muscles, including the chest, shoulders, and triceps, while also engaging secondary muscles such as the core, back, and legs for stability and support. By performing push-ups regularly, you can achieve a sculpted upper body and improve overall physical fitness.

How to Perform Push-Ups:

- Start in a plank position with your hands positioned slightly wider than shoulder-width apart and your body forming a straight line from head to heels.
- Engage your core muscles and lower your body by bending your elbows until your chest nearly touches the ground. Keep your elbows close to your sides throughout the movement.

- Push through your palms to straighten your arms and return to the starting position. Ensure that your body remains in a straight line throughout the exercise.
- Repeat for the desired number of repetitions, focusing on maintaining proper form and engaging the target muscles throughout the movement.

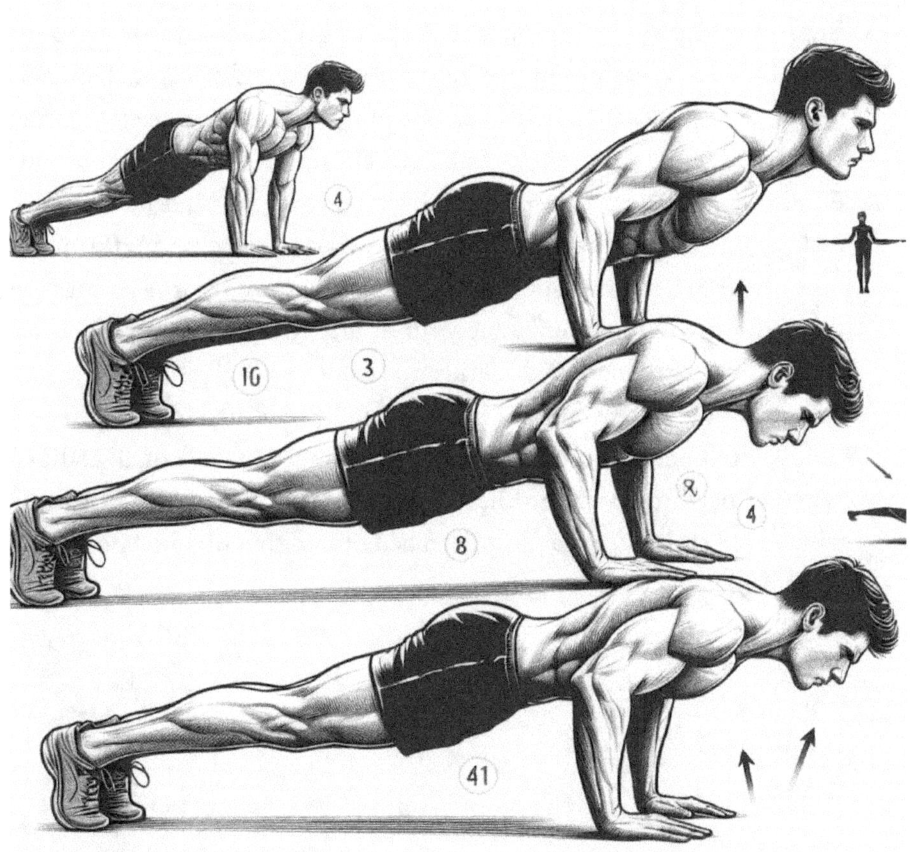

Key Benefits of Push-Ups:

1. Upper Body Strength: Push-ups are an excellent strength-building exercise for the muscles of the chest, shoulders, and arms. The pushing

motion engages these muscles, promoting muscle growth and increasing overall upper body strength.

2. Core Stability: Maintaining a plank-like position throughout the push-up exercise requires activation of the core muscles, including the abdominals and obliques, to stabilize the body. This helps improve core strength and stability, leading to better posture and reduced risk of back pain.

3. Improved Muscle Definition: Push-ups target multiple muscle groups simultaneously, including the chest, shoulders, and triceps. Regularly performing push-ups can help define and sculpt these muscles, giving your upper body a more toned and athletic appearance.

4. Functional Strength: Push-ups mimic real-life pushing movements, making them a functional exercise that translates to better performance in daily activities and sports. Developing strength and endurance through push-ups can enhance your ability to push objects, perform chores, and participate in athletic endeavors.

5. Versatility and Accessibility: Push-ups can be modified to suit different fitness levels and goals, making them accessible to people of all abilities. Whether performed on the knees, with incline or decline variations, or with added resistance, push-ups can be tailored to individual needs and preferences.

5

JUMP ROPE EXERCISE

4) Jump Rope Exercise

Jump rope, also known as skipping, is a dynamic and versatile cardiovascular exercise that offers numerous health and fitness benefits. This high-intensity workout requires minimal equipment and space, making it an ideal option for individuals looking to boost their fitness levels and burn calories effectively.

Jumping rope engages multiple muscle groups throughout the body, including the legs, core, arms, and shoulders, making it a full-body workout. In addition to improving cardiovascular health and endurance, jump rope exercises can enhance coordination, agility, and balance.

How to Perform Jump Rope:

- Begin by wearing comfortable athletic shoes with adequate cushioning and support to absorb impact.
- Hold the handles of a wire jump rope in each hand, allowing the rope to hang behind your body.
- Swing the rope over your head in a circular motion, bringing it down toward your feet as you jump off the ground.
- Time your jumps to coincide with the rotation of the rope, aiming to

clear it with each jump.

- Start with a comfortable pace and gradually increase the intensity and duration of your jump rope session as you build stamina and proficiency.
- Practice regularly to improve your jumping technique and coordination, aiming for at least 5 to 10 minutes of continuous jumping per session.

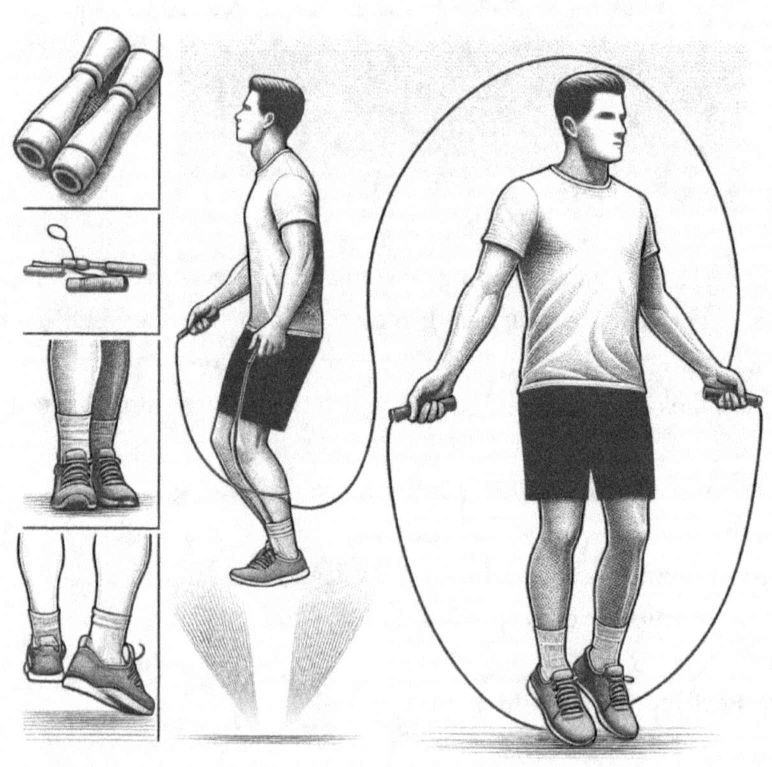

Key Benefits of Jump Rope:

1. Cardiovascular Health: Jumping rope elevates the heart rate, making it an effective aerobic exercise for improving cardiovascular health and

endurance. Regular jump rope sessions can help strengthen the heart, increase lung capacity, and lower the risk of cardiovascular diseases.

2. Calorie Burn and Weight Loss: Jump rope exercises are highly effective for burning calories and promoting weight loss. The combination of high-intensity cardio and full-body engagement can help torch calories and shed excess fat, particularly around the waist and abdominal area.

3. Muscle Toning and Strength: Jumping rope targets the muscles in the legs, including the calves, quadriceps, and hamstrings, as well as the core muscles, arms, and shoulders. The repetitive jumping motion helps tone and strengthen these muscle groups, leading to improved muscle definition and endurance.

4. Improved Coordination and Agility: Jump rope exercises require coordination and timing to execute the jumps accurately. Regular practice can enhance coordination, agility, and proprioception, which are essential for overall athletic performance and injury prevention.

5. Portability and Convenience: Jumping rope requires minimal equipment—a jump rope and a flat surface—making it a portable and convenient exercise option. It can be done virtually anywhere, whether at home, in the gym, or outdoors, making it accessible for individuals with busy lifestyles.

Incorporating jump rope exercises into your fitness routine can provide a fun and effective way to boost cardiovascular health, burn calories, and improve overall physical fitness. Whether used as a standalone workout or as part of a comprehensive training program, jumping rope offers a wide range of benefits for individuals of all fitness levels and ages.

6

BURPEE EXERCISE

5) Burpee Exercise

Burpees stand as a dynamic and challenging full-body exercise that combines elements of cardiovascular conditioning and strength training. This plyometric exercise (power exercise that is explosive and involves the stretching and contracting of muscles repeatedly) requires no equipment, making it a convenient and effective workout option for individuals seeking to enhance their fitness levels and burn calories efficiently.

Burpees engage multiple muscle groups throughout the body, including the upper body, lower body, and core, making it a comprehensive workout that targets strength, endurance, and agility. This high-intensity exercise can elevate the heart rate rapidly, providing cardiovascular benefits while also promoting muscle growth and toning.

How to Perform Burpees:

- Begin in a standing position with your feet shoulder-width apart on a flat surface.
- Lower your body into a squat position, bending at the knees and hips while keeping your back straight and chest lifted.

- Place your hands on the ground in front of you and jump your feet back into a plank position, maintaining a straight line from head to heels.
- Perform a push-up by lowering your chest to the ground while keeping your elbows close to your sides.
- Push through your palms to return to the plank position, then jump your feet forward toward your hands, landing softly in a squat position.
- Explosively jump upward, extending your arms overhead as you propel yourself off the ground.
- Land as softly as you can and immediately lower back again into the squat position to repeat the process.

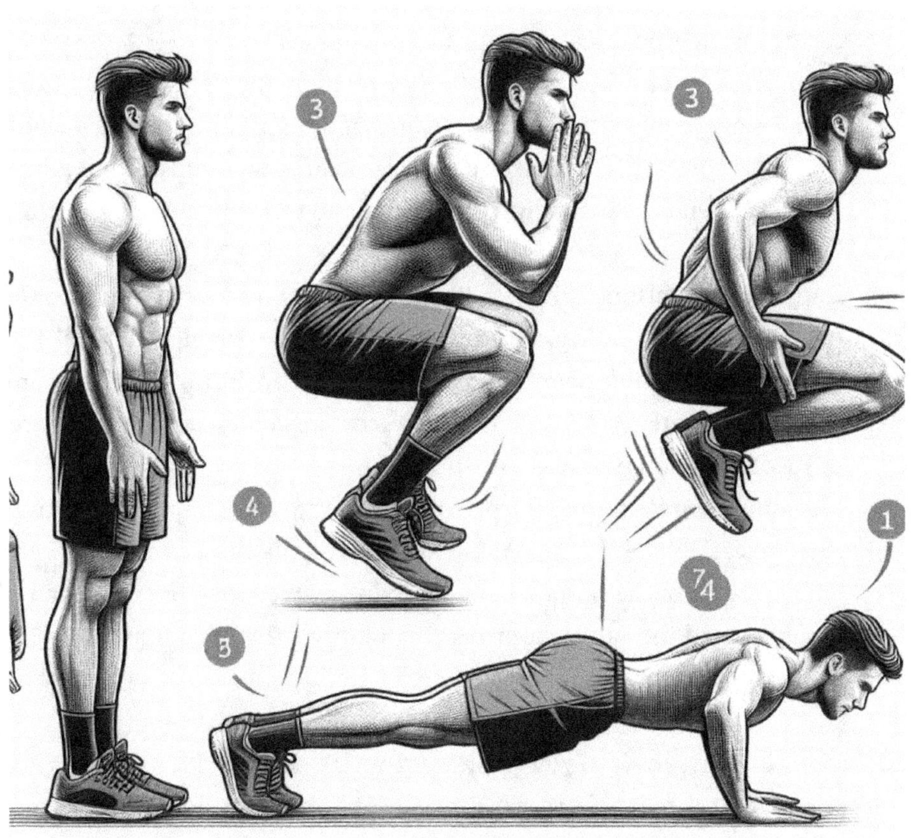

Key Benefits of Burpees:

1. Full-Body Workout: Burpees target a wide range of muscle groups, including the chest, shoulders, arms, back, core, glutes, quadriceps, and hamstrings. By engaging multiple muscle groups simultaneously, burpees provide a comprehensive full-body workout that improves strength, endurance, and muscular coordination.

2. Cardiovascular Conditioning: Burpees are an effective cardiovascular exercise that elevates the heart rate and promotes efficient calorie burning. The rapid succession of movements, including jumping, squatting, and push-ups, challenges the cardiovascular system, improving overall cardiovascular health and endurance.

3. Calorie Burn and Weight Loss: Due to their high-intensity nature, burpees are highly effective for burning calories and promoting weight loss. This compound exercise engages large muscle groups and requires significant energy expenditure, making it an efficient calorie-burning workout.

4. Improved Functional Fitness: Burpees mimic functional movements like squatting, jumping, and push-ups, making them beneficial for improving overall functional fitness and athletic performance. By enhancing strength, agility, and power, burpees can improve performance in sports and activities of daily living.

5. No Equipment Required: Burpees require no special equipment, making them accessible and convenient for individuals to perform virtually anywhere. Whether at home, in the gym, or outdoors, burpees can be incorporated into a workout routine without the need for expensive equipment or gym memberships.

Incorporating burpees into your workout routine can provide a challenging and effective way to improve cardiovascular fitness, build strength, and enhance overall physical conditioning. By performing burpees with proper form and intensity, you can maximize the benefits of this versatile exercise for achieving your fitness goals.

7

BREATHING EXERCISE

6) Breathing Exercise

Engaging in deliberate breathing exercises can profoundly impact both physical and mental well-being:

How to Perform Breathing Exercise:

- Inhale slowly, counting silently from 1 to 5 as you fill your lungs with air.
- Hold your breath, maintaining that count of 1 to 5 in your mind, allowing the oxygen to circulate through your body.
- Then, exhale gently, counting again from 1 to 5, releasing any tension or stress with each breath. Repeat this cycle for a duration of 10 minutes.

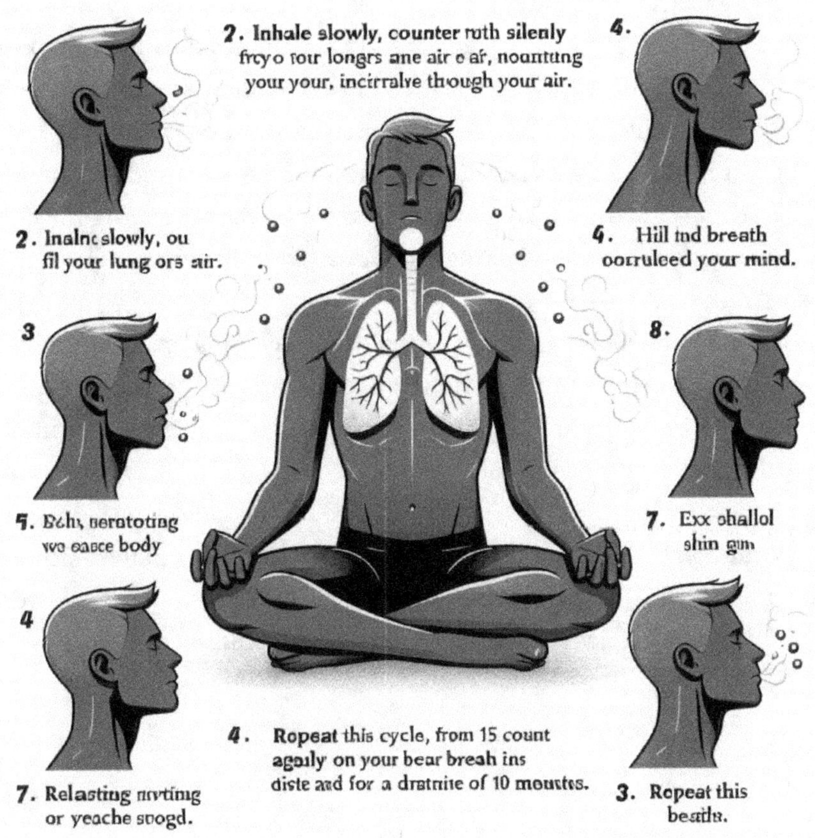

Benefits of Breathing Exercise:

1. Stress Reduction: By triggering the body's relaxation response, deep breathing aids in the reduction of stress hormones like cortisol, fostering a sense of calmness and tranquility.

2. Anxiety Management: Deep breathing techniques can effectively alleviate symptoms of anxiety by inducing relaxation and diminishing physiological arousal, providing relief from feelings of tension or unease.

3. Enhanced Focus and Concentration: By directing attention to the counting and rhythm of breath, this exercise can quiet the mind and cultivate mindfulness, fostering improved focus and concentration

during tasks or activities.

4. Improved Oxygenation: Deep breathing facilitates the intake of oxygen-rich air, optimizing oxygenation of the blood and tissues. This can lead to heightened energy levels and a renewed sense of vitality.

5. Lowered Blood Pressure: The relaxation response induced by deep breathing aids in reducing blood pressure levels, mitigating the body's stress response and benefiting individuals with hypertension or cardiovascular issues.

6. Better Sleep Quality: Incorporating deep breathing exercises into your bedtime routine can promote relaxation and ease the transition into sleep, potentially enhancing the overall quality of sleep and promoting feelings of restfulness upon waking.

Incorporating regular deep breathing practices into your daily routine can yield a multitude of benefits for both physical and mental health, fostering relaxation, stress management, and overall well-being.

8

WALKING LUNGES

7) Walking Lunges:

Description: Walking lunges are a dynamic lower body exercise that targets the quadriceps, hamstrings, glutes, and calves.

How to Perform Walking Lunges:

- Stand with your feet hip-width apart.
- Take a large step forward with your right foot, lowering your body until both knees are bent at 90-degree angles.
- Keep your chest up and your front knee aligned with your ankle.
- Push through your front heel to return to the starting position, then repeat with the left leg.
- Continue alternating legs as you walk forward.

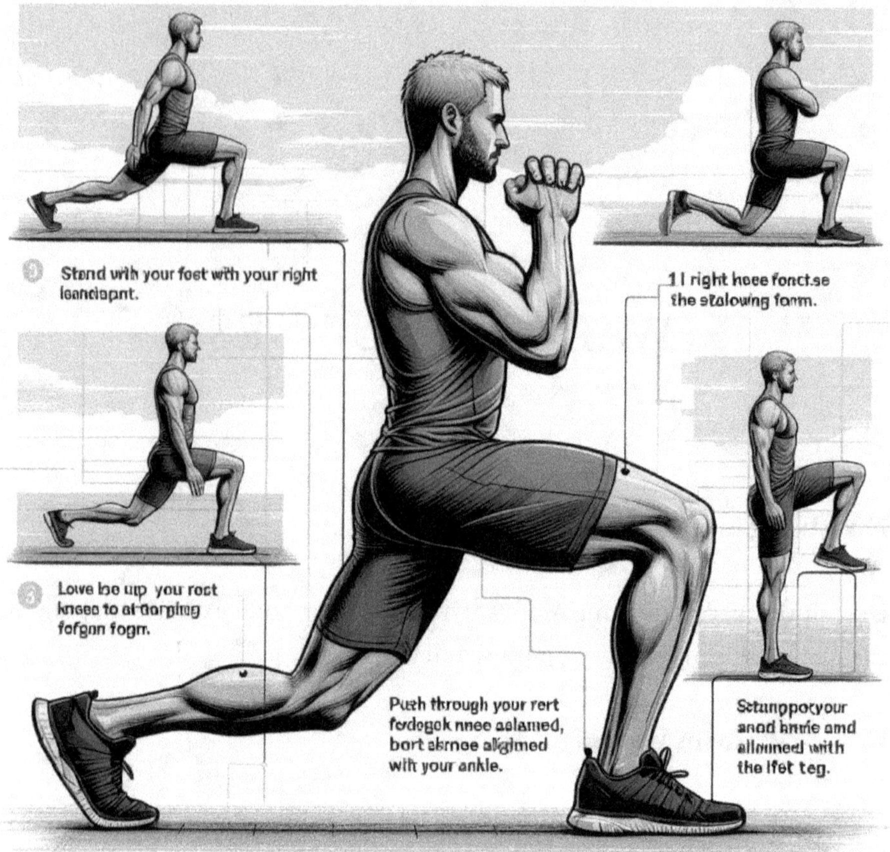

Benefits of Walking Lunges:

1. Strengthens lower body muscles.
2. Improves balance and coordination.
3. Enhances hip flexibility.
4. Provides cardiovascular benefits when done at a brisk pace.

Incorporating these simple exercises into your workout routine can help you build strength, improve mobility, and enhance overall physical fitness. Plus, they require minimal equipment and can be easily modified to suit your fitness level and goals.

9

JUMPING JACKS EXERCISE

8) Jumping Jacks:

Description: Jumping jacks are a dynamic cardiovascular exercise that engages the entire body and elevates the heart rate.

How to Perform Jumping Jacks:

- Start with your feet together and your arms at your sides.
- Jump explosively, spreading your legs wide and raising your arms overhead.
- Quickly return to the starting position by jumping back to the feet together and lowering your arms to your sides.
- Repeat this motion continuously for a set duration or number of repetitions.

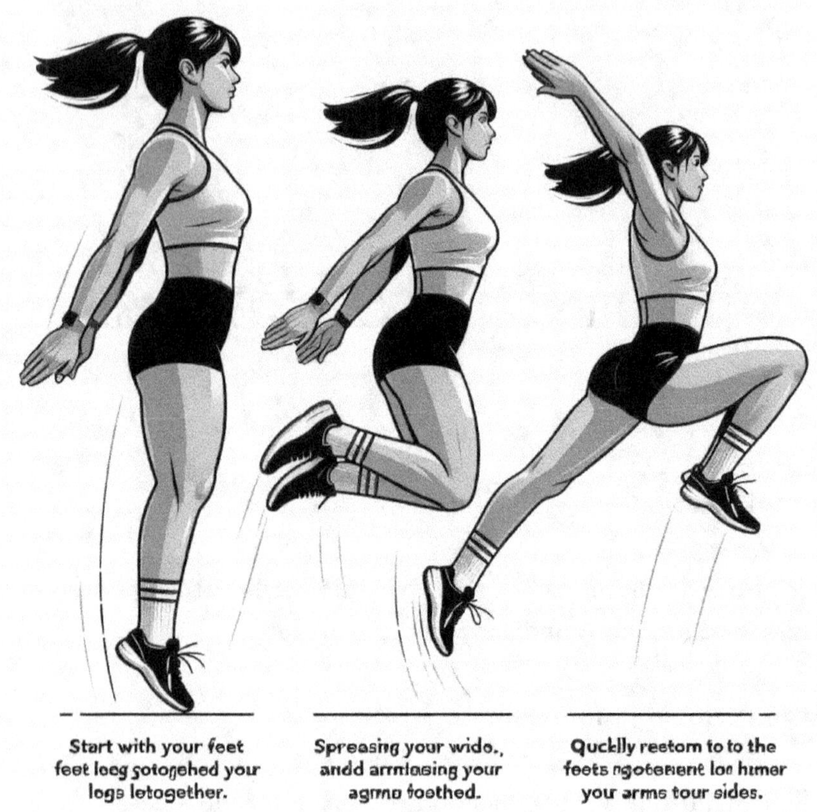

Benefits of Jumping Jacks:

1. Improves cardiovascular health and endurance.
2. Burns calories and promotes weight loss.
3. Increases coordination and agility.
4. Requires no equipment and can be done anywhere.

10

BICYCLE CRUNCHES EXERCISE

9) Bicycle Crunches:

Description: Bicycle crunches are an effective abdominal exercise that targets the rectus abdominis and obliques.

How to Perform Bicycle Crunches:

- Lie on your back with your hands positioned behind your head, and elevate your legs while bending your knees at a 90-degree angle..
- Alternate bringing your right elbow towards your left knee while straightening your right leg, then switch sides, bringing your left elbow towards your right knee.
- Continue alternating sides in a pedaling motion, engaging your core throughout.
- Aim for 10-15 repetitions on each side.

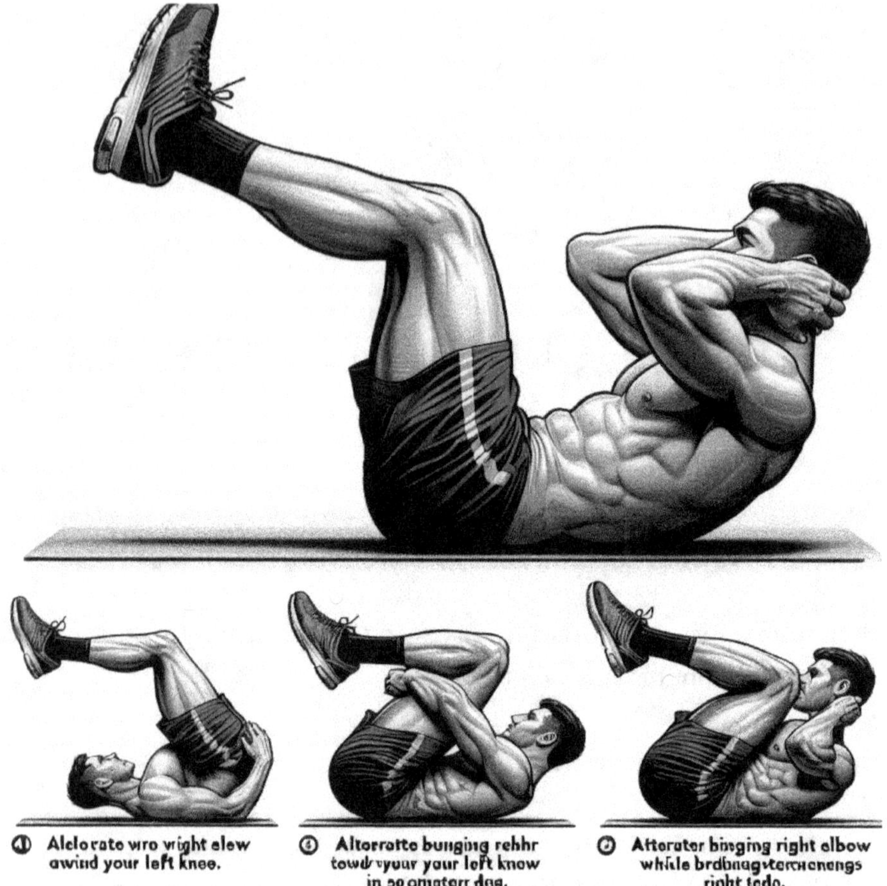

Benefits of Bicycle Crunches:

1. Strengthens abdominal muscles.
2. Targets both upper and lower abs.
3. Improves core stability and coordination.
4. Can be modified for different fitness levels.

11

RUSSIAN TWISTS EXERCISE

10) Russian Twists:

Description: Russian twists are a core-strengthening exercise that targets the obliques and lower back muscles.

How to Perform Russian Twists:

- Sit comfortably on the floor with your knees bent and your feet flat on the ground.
- Lean back slightly, keeping your back straight and your core engaged.
- Hold a weight or medicine ball with both hands, or clasp your hands together.
- Twist your torso to the right, bringing the weight or hands towards the floor beside your hip.
- Return to the center, then twist to the left, alternating sides in a controlled motion.
- Aim for 10-15 repetitions on each side.

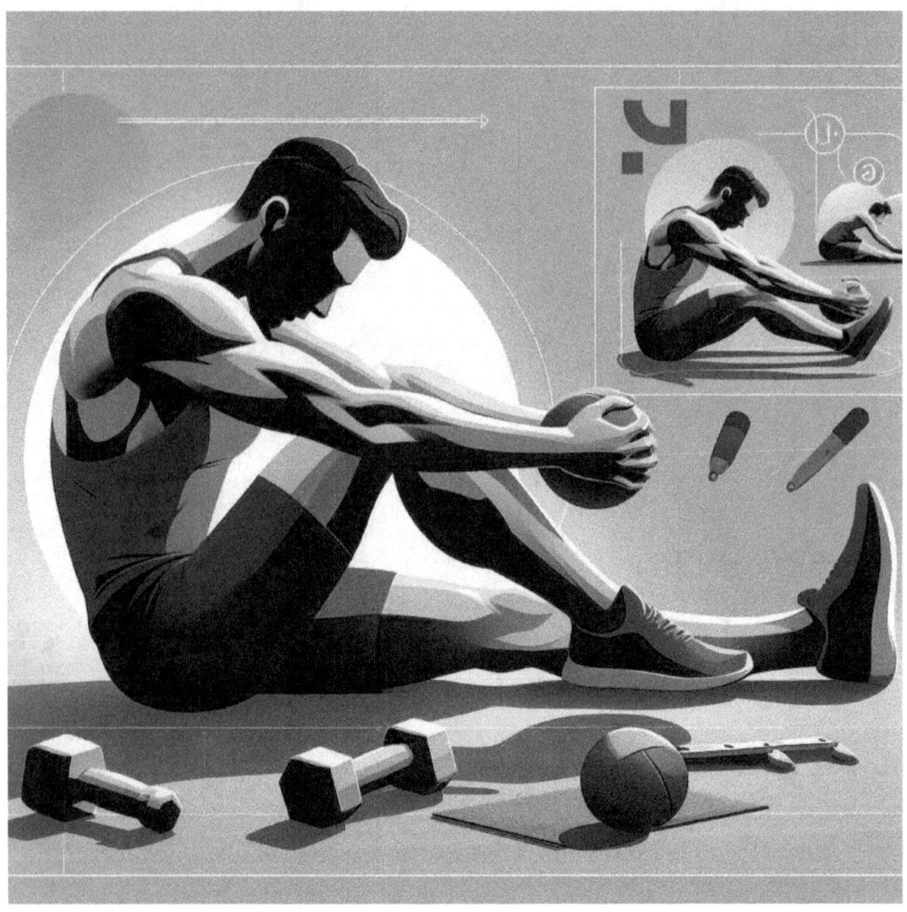

Benefits of Russian Twists:

1. Targets oblique muscles.
2. Improves rotational strength and mobility.
3. Enhances core stability and balance.
4. Can be performed with or without weights.

12

MOUNTAIN CLIMBERS EXERCISE

11) Mountain Climbers:

Description: Mountain climbers are a dynamic full-body exercise that targets the core, shoulders, arms, and legs.

How to Perform Mountain Climbers:

- Start in a push-up position, with your hands directly under your shoulders and your body forming a straight line from head to heels.
- Engage your core muscles and bring one knee towards your chest,
- Then quickly switch legs, jumping to bring the other knee towards your chest.
- Continue alternating legs in a running motion, keeping your hips level and your core engaged throughout.
- Aim for 20-30 seconds of continuous movement.

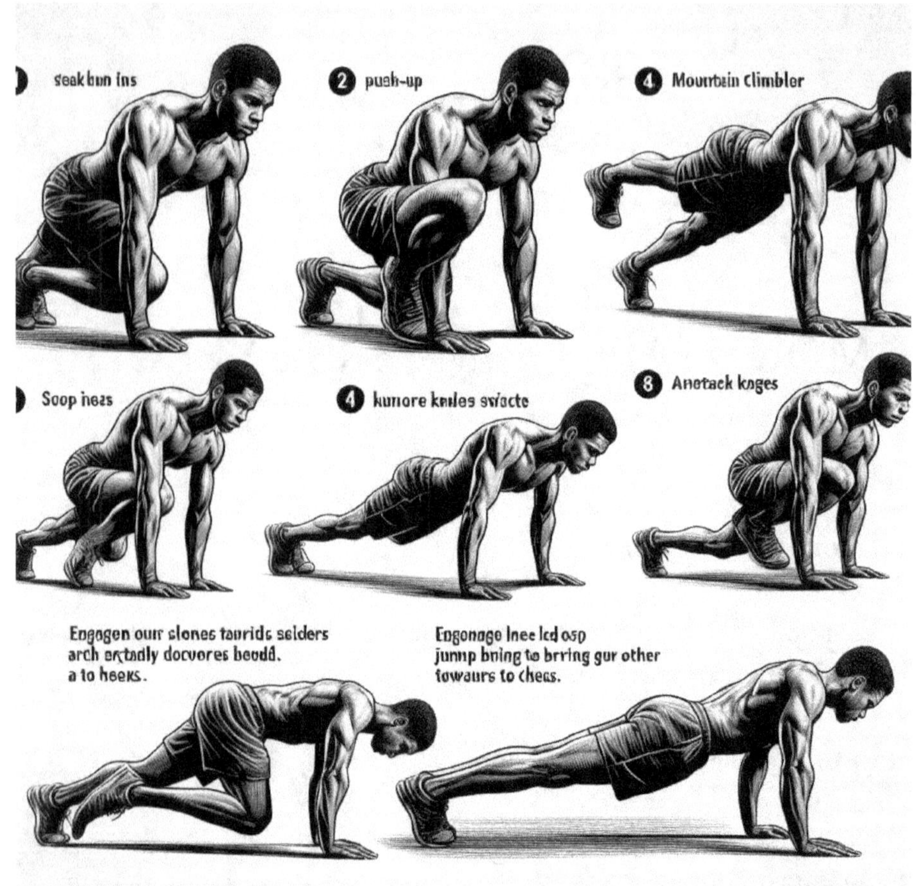

Benefits of Mountain Climbers:

1. Elevates heart rate for cardiovascular benefits.
2. Strengthens core muscles.
3. Improves coordination and agility.
4. Requires no equipment and can be done anywhere.

13

TRICEP DIPS EXERCISE

12) Tricep Dips:

Description: Tricep dips are a bodyweight exercise that targets the muscles of the triceps, shoulders, and chest.

How to Perform Tricep Dips:

- Take a seat on the front edge of a stable chair or bench, positioning your hands shoulder-width apart beside your hips.
- Extend your legs in front of you with your heels on the ground.
- Lift your hips off the chair and walk your feet forward slightly.
- Bend your elbows to lower your body towards the ground, keeping your back close to the chair.
- Press through your palms to straighten your arms and return to the starting position.
- Aim for 10-15 repetitions.

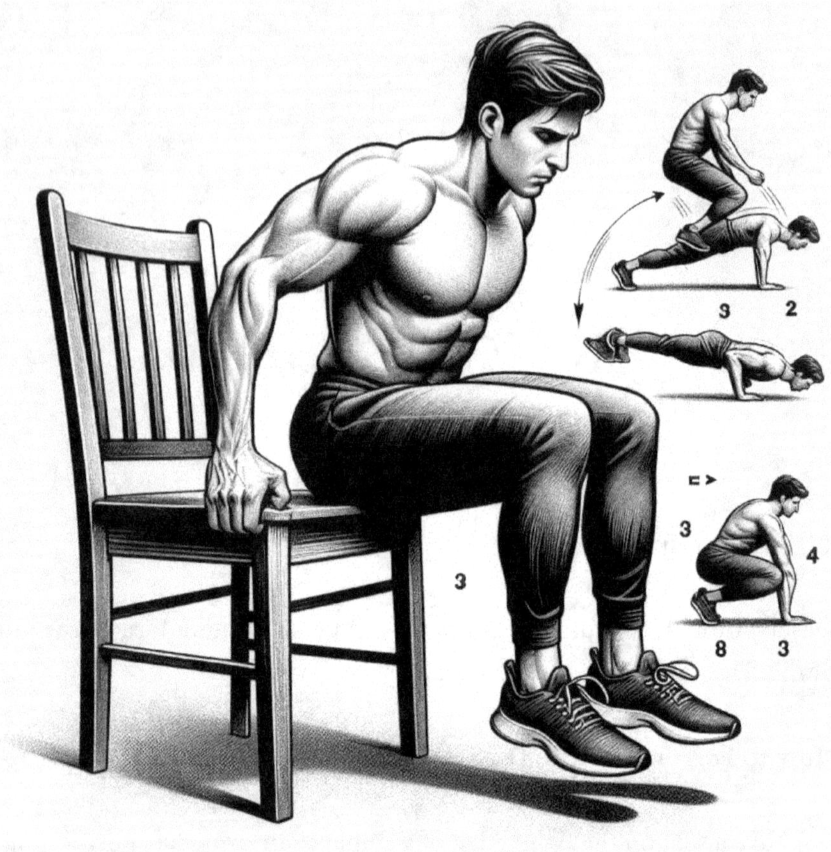

Benefits of Tricep Dips:

1. Targets tricep muscles.
2. Improves upper body strength and tone.
3. Enhances shoulder stability.
4. Can be performed with minimal equipment.

14

SIDE PLANK

13) Side Plank:

Description: The side plank is a variation of the plank exercise that targets the muscles of the core, particularly the obliques.

How to Perform Side Plank:

- Start by lying on your side with your legs straight and your elbow directly under your shoulder.
- Lift your hips off the ground, forming a straight line from head to heels.
- Engage your core muscles and hold this position for 20-30 seconds.
- Repeat on the other side, balancing on your opposite elbow and lifting your hips off the ground.
- Aim for 2-3 sets on each side.

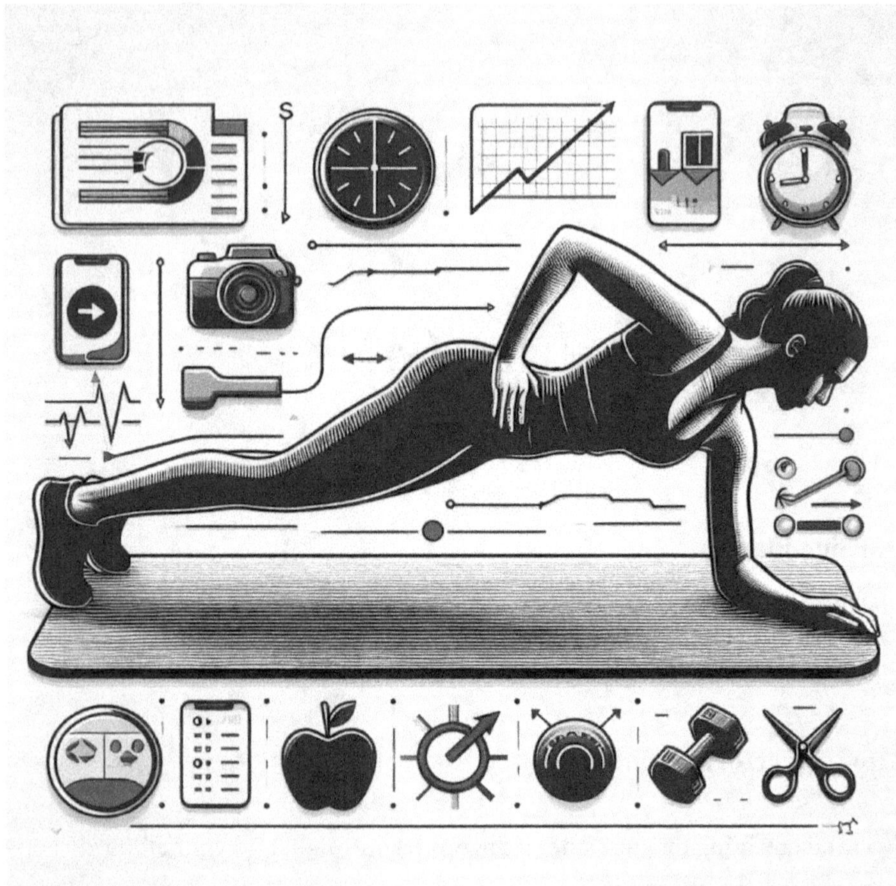

Benefits of Side Plank:

- Strengthens oblique muscles.
- Improves lateral stability and balance.
- Enhances core strength and endurance.
- Can be modified for different fitness levels.

15

SUPERMAN EXERCISE

14) Superman Exercise:

Description: The Superman exercise targets the muscles of the lower back, glutes, and hamstrings, promoting spinal stability and strength.

How to Perform Superman Exercise:

- Lie face down on the ground with your arms extended overhead and your legs straight.
- Engage your core muscles and lift your arms, chest, and legs off the ground simultaneously.
- Hold this position for 3-5 seconds, then lower back down to the starting position.
- Aim for 10-15 repetitions.

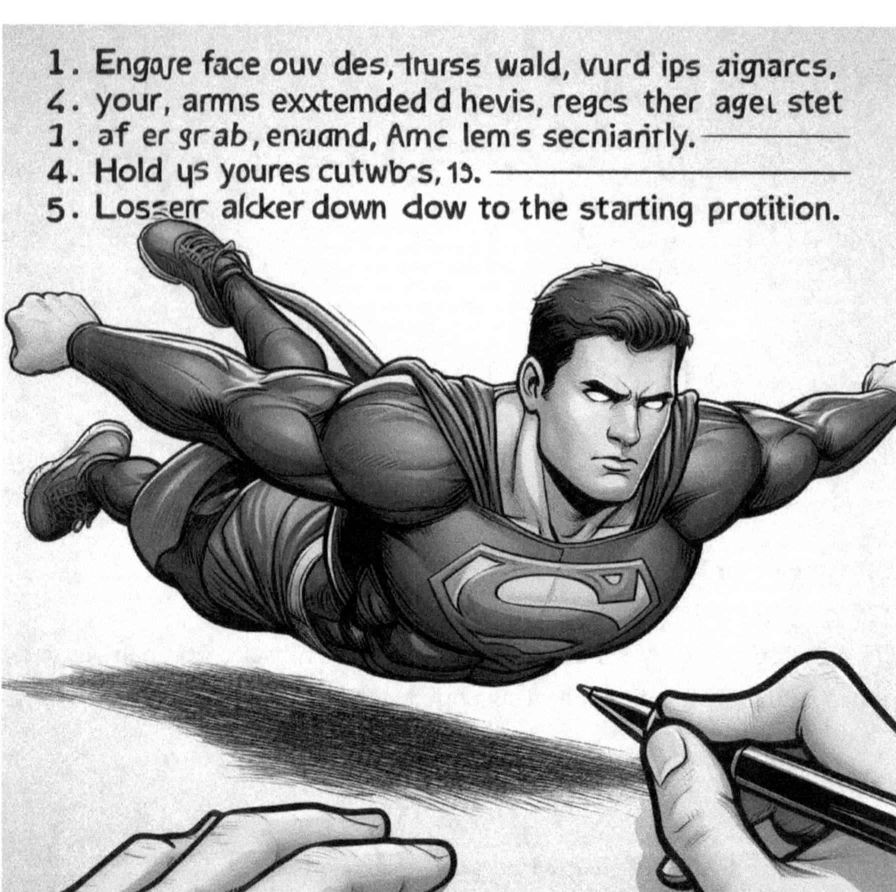

Benefits of Superman Exercise:

1. Strengthens lower back muscles.
2. Improves spinal stability and posture.
3. Targets glutes and hamstrings.
4. Can help alleviate lower back pain.

16

STANDING CALF RAISES EXERCISE

15) Standing Calf Raises:

Description: Standing calf raises target the muscles of the calves, specifically the gastrocnemius and soleus.

How to Perform Standing Calf Raises:

- Stand with your feet hip-width apart and your hands resting on a stable surface for support.
- Lift your heels off the ground as high as possible, rising onto the balls of your feet.
- Hold the top position for 1-2 seconds, then lower back down to the starting position.
- Aim for 15-20 repetitions.

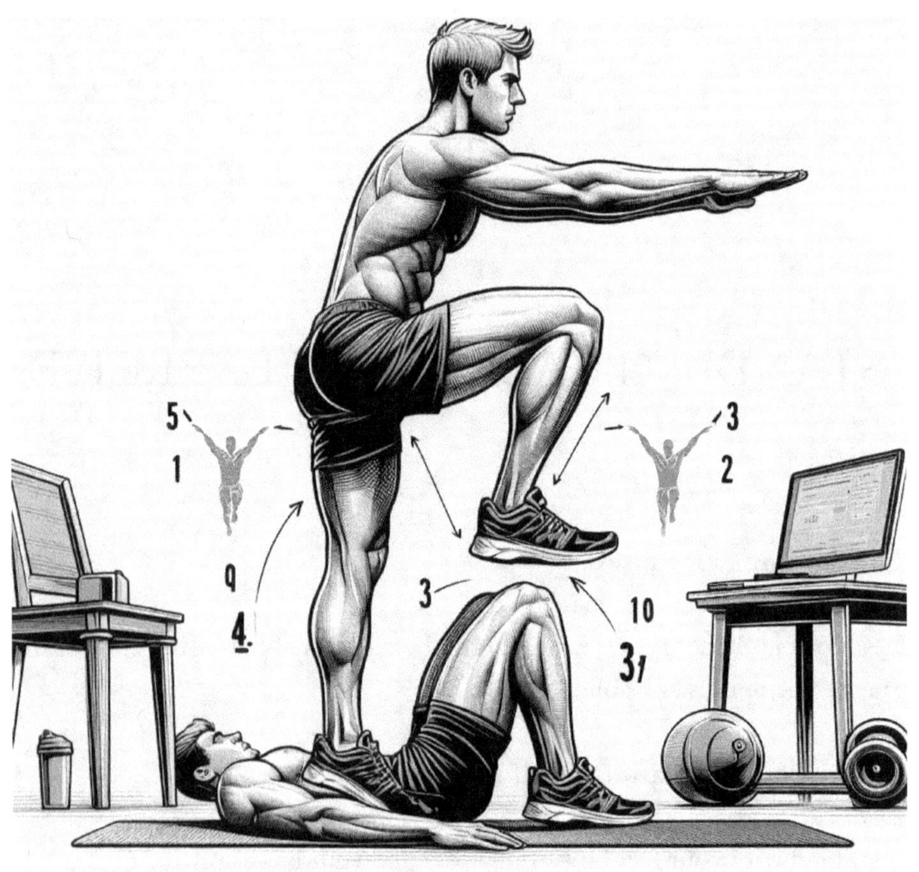

Benefits of Standing Calf Raises:

1. Strengthens calf muscles.
2. Improves ankle stability and balance.
3. Enhances lower body strength and power.
4. Can be performed anywhere with minimal equipment.

WALL SIT EXERCISE

16) Wall Sit:

Description: The wall sit is a static lower body exercise that targets the quadriceps, hamstrings, and glutes.

How to Perform Wall Sit:

- Stand with your back against a sturdy wall and your feet shoulder-width apart.
- Slide your back down the wall until your thighs are parallel to the ground, forming a seated position.
- Hold this position for 30-60 seconds, keeping your back flat against the wall and your knees at a 90-degree angle.
- Aim for 2-3 sets.

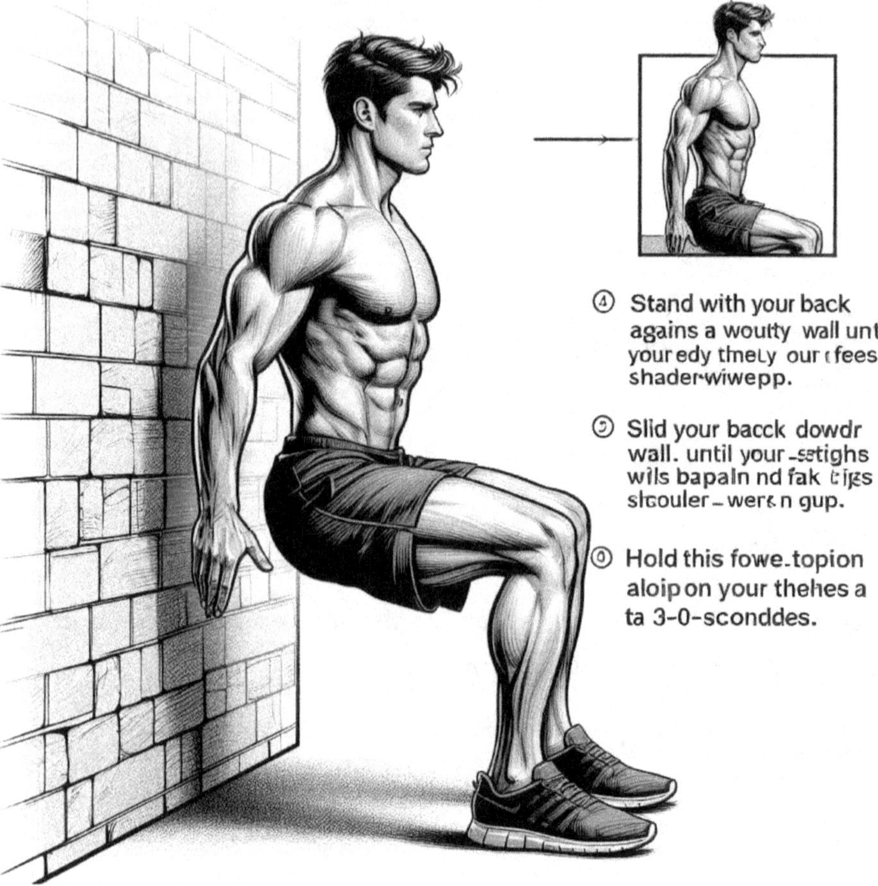

Benefits of Wall Sit:

1. Strengthens lower body muscles.
2. Improves muscular endurance.
3. Enhances quadriceps and glute activation.
4. Can be done anywhere with a wall for support.

18

LATERAL LUNGES EXERCISE

17) Lateral Lunges:

Description: Lateral lunges target the muscles of the inner and outer thighs, glutes, and hips.

How to Perform Lateral Lunges:

- Stand with your feet together and your hands on your hips.
- Take a large step to the side with your right foot, keeping your left leg straight.
- Bend your right knee and push your hips back, lowering your body towards the ground.
- Keep your chest up and your left leg straight as you lunge to the side.
- Push through your right heel to return to the starting position, then repeat on the left side.
- Aim for 10-12 repetitions on each side.

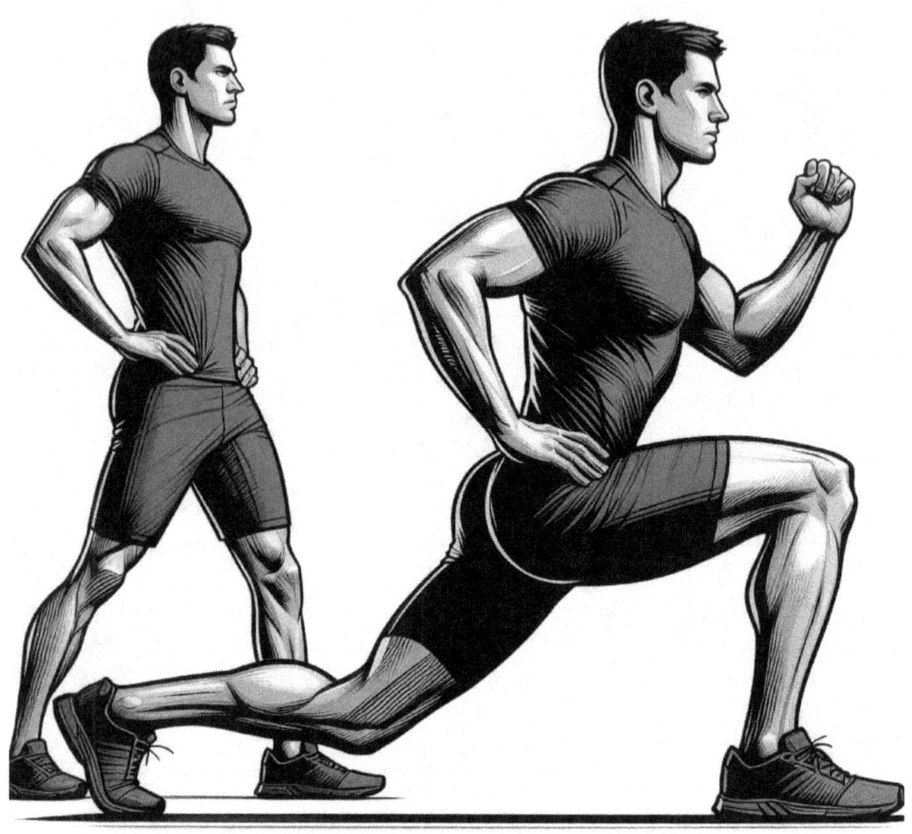

Benefits of Lateral Lunges:

1. Targets inner and outer thigh muscles.
2. Improves hip mobility and flexibility.
3. Enhances lateral stability and balance.
4. Can be performed with or without weights.

19

SINGLE-LEG GLUTE BRIDGE EXERCISE

18) Single-Leg Glute Bridge:

Description: The single-leg glute bridge targets the glutes, hamstrings, and lower back, while also improving hip stability.

How to Perform Single-Leg Glute Bridge:

- Lie on your back with your knees bent and your feet flat on the ground.
- Extend one leg straight up towards the ceiling, keeping the other foot flat on the ground.
- Press through the heel of the grounded foot to lift your hips towards the ceiling, squeezing your glutes at the top.
- Lower your hips back down to the ground with control, then repeat on the other side.
- Aim for 10-12 repetitions on each leg.

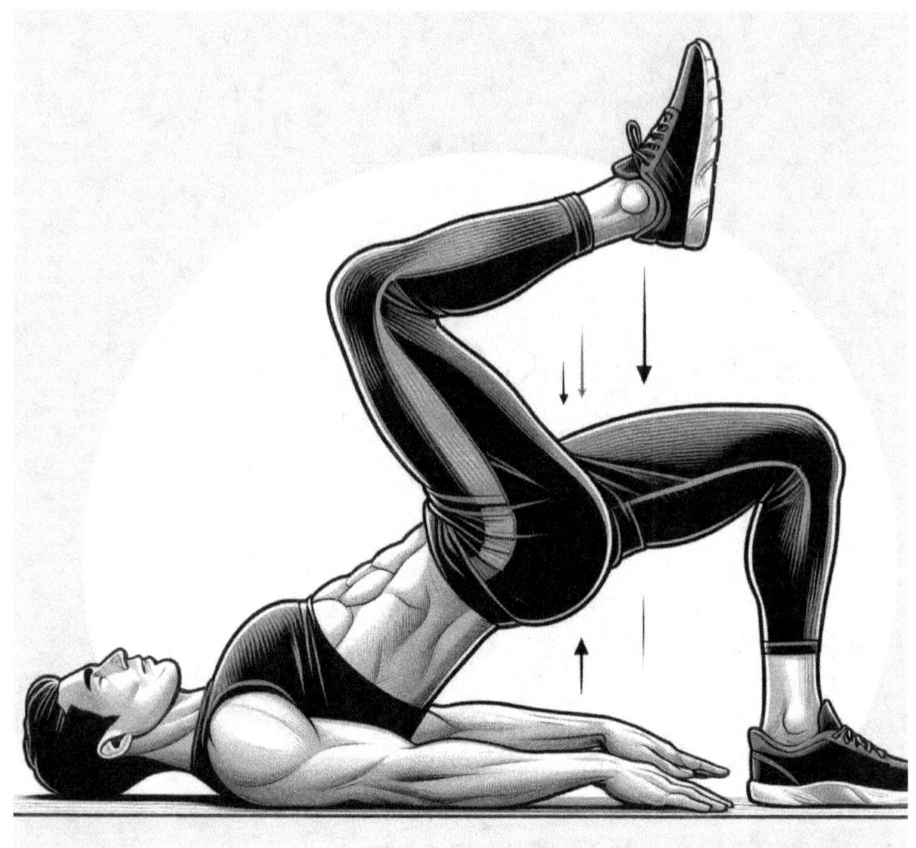

Benefits of Single-Leg Glute Bridge:

1. Strengthens glute muscles.
2. Improves hip stability and mobility.
3. Targets hamstrings and lower back muscles.
4. Can help prevent lower body imbalances and injuries.

20

HIGH KNEES EXERCISE

19) High Knees:

Description: High knees are a dynamic cardiovascular exercise that elevates the heart rate and engages the muscles of the legs and core.

How to Perform High Knees:

- Stand with your feet hip-width apart and your arms at your sides.
- Quickly lift one knee towards your chest as high as possible, then switch legs, alternating knees in a running motion.
- Pump your arms in coordination with your legs, keeping a fast pace to elevate your heart rate.
- Aim for 30-60 seconds of continuous movement.

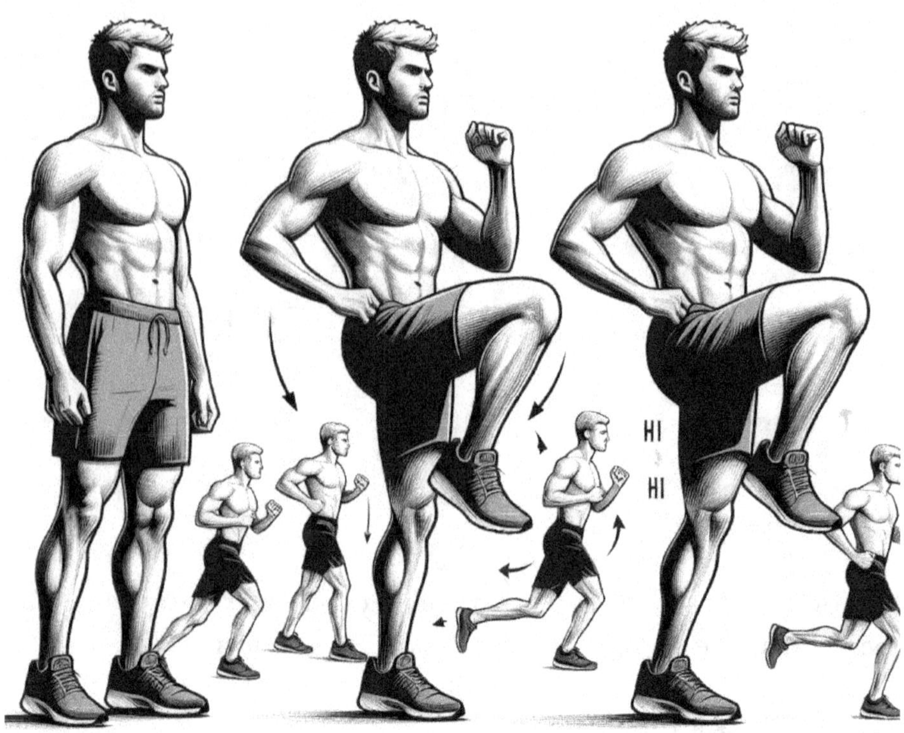

Benefits of High Knees:

1. Elevates heart rate for cardiovascular benefits.
2. Improves lower body strength and coordination.
3. Engages core muscles for stability and balance.
4. Requires no equipment and can be done anywhere.

21

BIRD DOG EXERCISE

20) Bird Dog Exercise:

Description: The bird dog exercise targets the muscles of the core, including the abdominals, lower back, and glutes.

How to Perform Bird Dog Exercise:

- Start on your hands and knees in a tabletop position, with your wrists aligned under your shoulders and your knees under your hips.
- Extend your right arm forward and your left leg back, keeping your hips level and your back flat.
- Hold this position for a few seconds, then return to the starting position and repeat on the other side.
- Aim for 10-12 repetitions on each side.

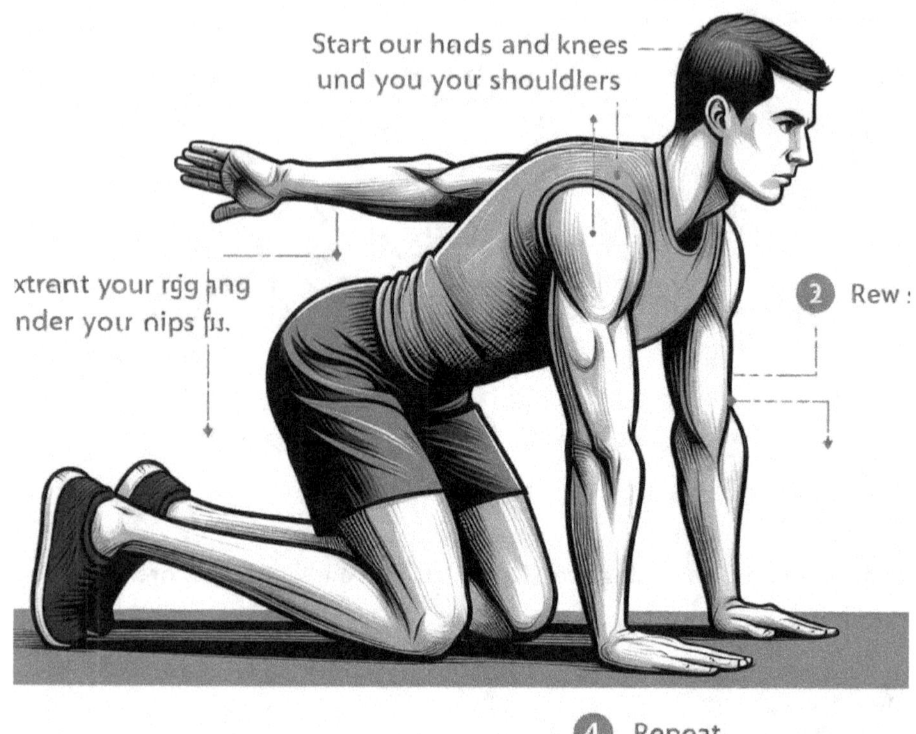

Benefits of Bird Dog Exercise:

1. Strengthens core muscles.
2. Improves balance and stability.
3. Targets lower back and glute muscles.
4. Can help prevent lower back pain and improve posture.

22

ORDINARY LEG RAISES EXERCISE

21) Ordinary Leg Raises:

Description: Leg raises target the muscles of the lower abdominals, hip flexors, and lower back.

How to Perform Ordinary Leg Raises:

- Lie on your back with your legs straight and your arms at your sides.
- Lift your legs off the ground, keeping them straight and together, until they are perpendicular to the ground.
- Lower your legs back down towards the ground with control, stopping just before they touch the floor.
- Lift your legs back up to the starting position, using your core muscles to control the movement.
- Aim for 10-12 repetitions.

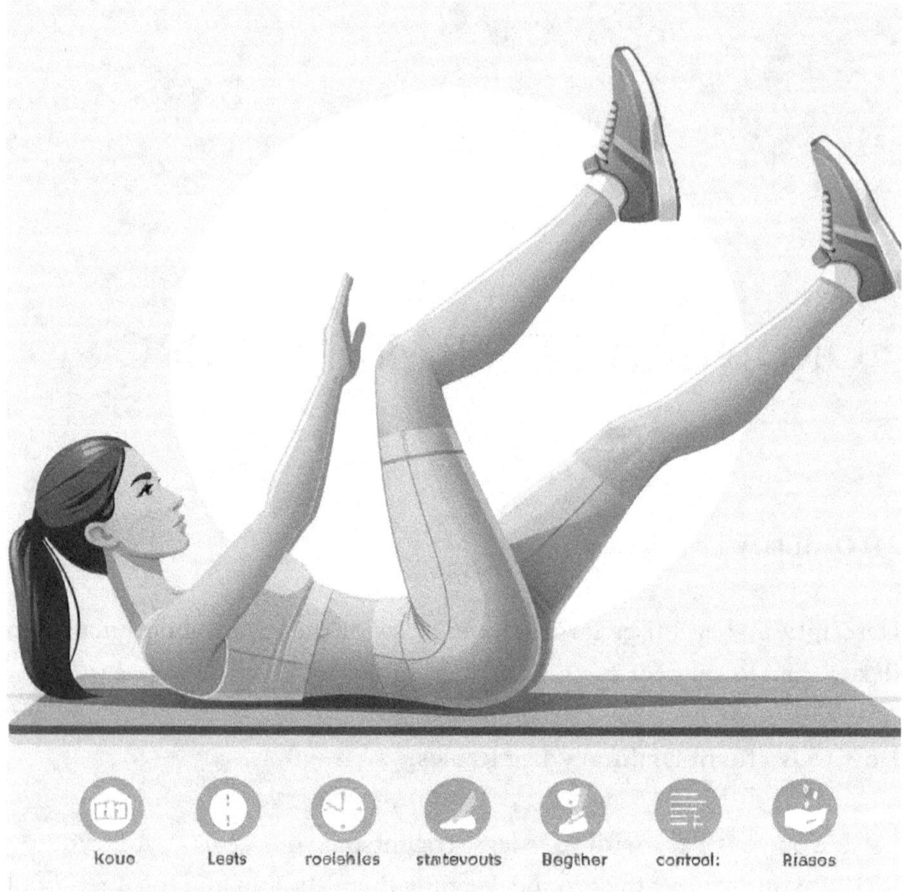

Benefits of Ordinary Leg Raises:

1. Targets lower abdominal muscles.
2. Strengthens hip flexors and lower back.
3. Improves core stability and control.
4. Can be performed with minimal equipment.

23

SIDE LEG RAISES EXERCISE

22) Side Leg Raises:

Description: Side leg raises target the muscles of the outer thighs, hips, and glutes.

How to Perform of Side Leg Raises:

- Lie on your side with your legs straight and your bottom arm extended under your head for support.
- Lift your top leg towards the ceiling as high as possible, keeping it straight and in line with your body.
- Lower your leg back down with control, stopping just before it touches the ground.
- Lift your leg back up to the starting position, using your outer thigh muscles to control the movement.
- Aim for 10-12 repetitions on each side.

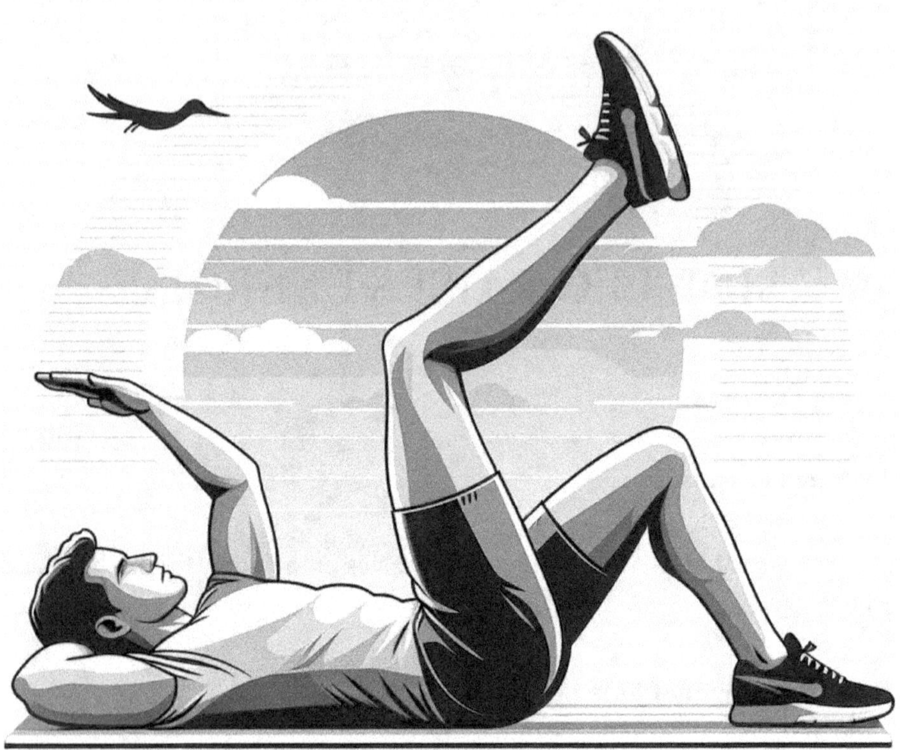

Benefits of Side Leg Raises:

1. Targets outer thigh muscles.
2. Strengthens hip abductors and glutes.
3. Improves hip stability and balance.
4. Can help prevent knee and hip injuries.

24

STANDING SHOULDER PRESS

23) Standing Shoulder Press:

Description: The standing shoulder press targets the muscles of the shoulders, arms, and upper back.

How to Perform Standing Shoulder Press:

- Stand with your feet hip-width apart and hold a dumbbell in each hand at shoulder height, palms facing forward.
- Press the weights overhead until your arms are fully extended, keeping your core engaged and your back straight.
- Lower the weights back down to shoulder height with control, then repeat for the desired number of repetitions.
- Aim for 10-12 repetitions.

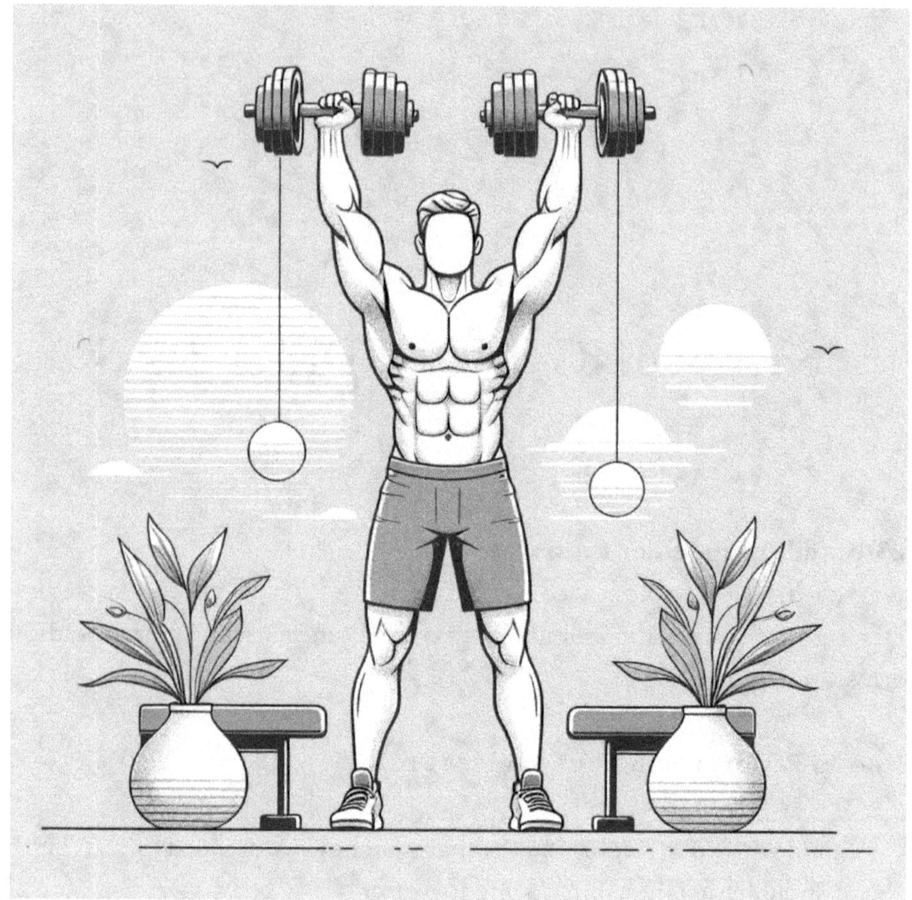

Benefits of Standing Shoulder Press:

1. Targets shoulder muscles (deltoids).
2. Strengthens arm muscles (triceps).
3. Improves upper body strength and tone.
4. Can be performed with dumbbells or resistance bands.

25

DEAD BUG EXERCISE

24) Dead Bug Exercise:

Description: The dead bug exercise is a core-strengthening movement that targets the abdominals and stabilizing muscles.

How to Perform Dead Bug Exercise:

- Lie on your back with your arms extended towards the ceiling and your legs lifted, knees bent at a 90-degree angle.
- Lower your right arm and left leg towards the ground, keeping them hovering just above the floor.
- Return to the starting position, then lower your left arm and right leg towards the ground.
- Continue alternating sides in a controlled manner, engaging your core throughout.
- Aim for 10-12 repetitions on each side.

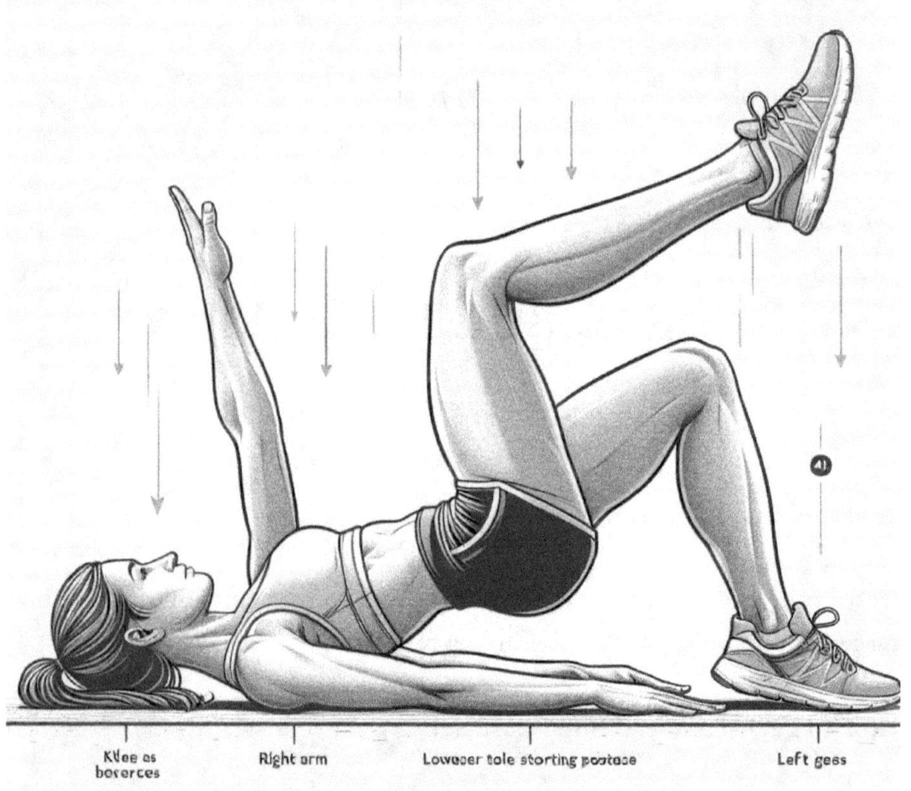

Benefits of Dead Bug Exercise:

1. Strengthens core muscles.
2. Improves coordination and stability.
3. Targets deep abdominal muscles.
4. Can help alleviate lower back pain.

26

PLANK WITH SHOULDER EXERCISE

25) Plank with Shoulder Taps:

Description: Plank with shoulder taps is a challenging variation of the traditional plank exercise that targets the core and shoulder stabilizers.

How to Perform Plank with Shoulder Taps:

- Start in a plank position with your hands directly under your shoulders and your body forming a straight line from head to heels.
- Keeping your hips stable, lift one hand off the ground and tap the opposite shoulder.
- Return to the starting position, then repeat on the other side.
- Continue alternating sides, keeping your core engaged to prevent rotation.
- Aim for 10-12 taps on each shoulder.

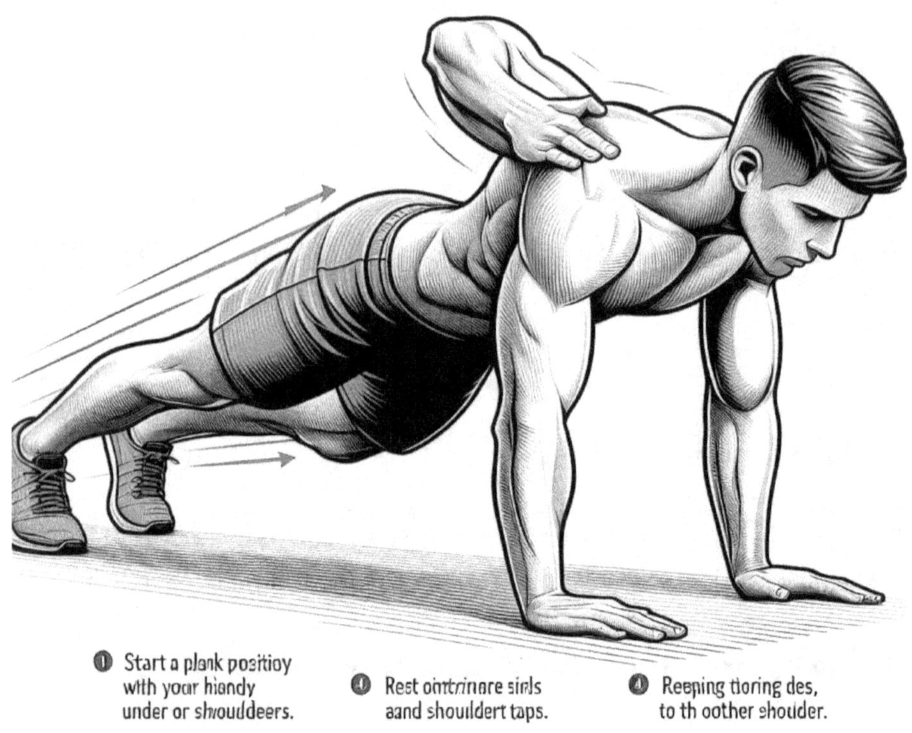

Benefits of Plank with Shoulder Taps:

1. Strengthens core muscles.
2. Improves shoulder stability and strength.
3. Enhances coordination and balance.
4. Increases intensity of traditional plank exercise.

27

REVERSE LUNGES EXERCISE

26) Reverse Lunges:

Description: Reverse lunges are a lower body exercise that targets the quadriceps, hamstrings, and glutes.

How to Perform Reverse Lunges:

- Stand with your feet hip-width apart and your hands on your hips.
- Step back with your right foot and lower your body until both knees are bent at 90-degree angles.
- Keep your chest up and your weight in your front heel.
- Push through your front heel to return to the starting position, then repeat on the other side.
- Aim for 10-12 repetitions on each leg.

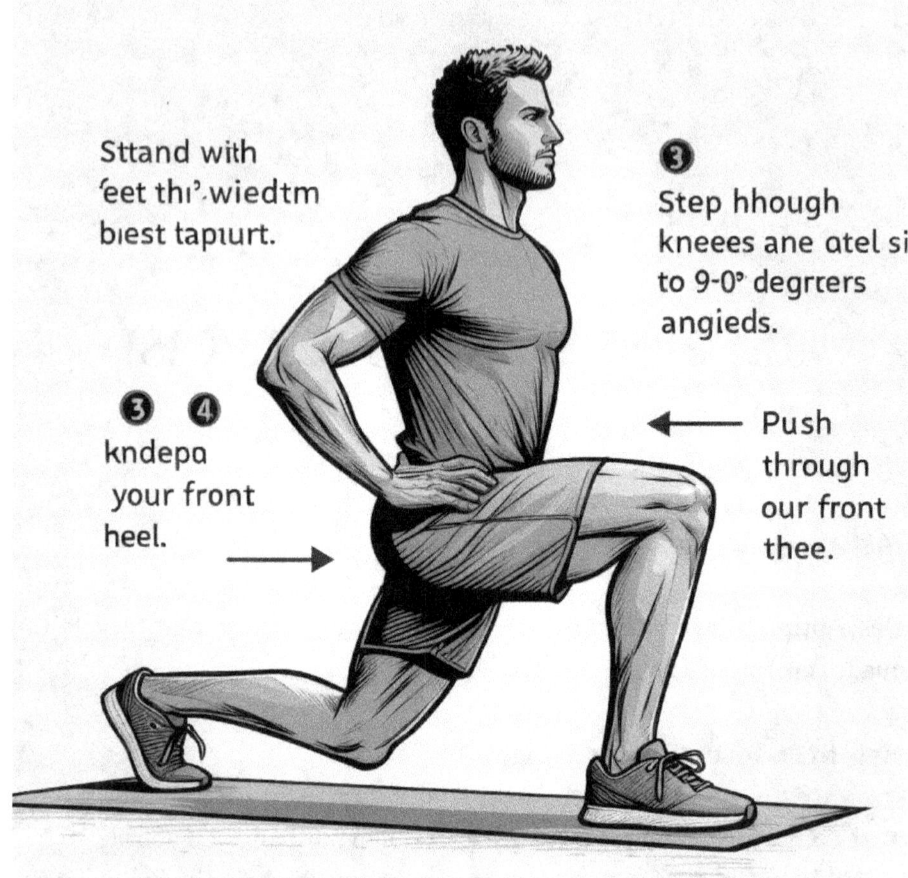

Benefits of Reverse Lunges:

1. Strengthens lower body muscles.
2. Improves balance and stability.
3. Targets glutes and hamstrings.
4. Reduces stress on knees compared to forward lunges.

28

SEATED LEG RAISES EXERCISE

27) Seated Leg Raises:

Description: Seated leg raises target the muscles of the lower abdominals and hip flexors.

How to Perform Seated Leg Raises:

- Sit on the edge of a sturdy chair or bench with your hands gripping the sides for support.
- Lean back slightly and lift your legs off the ground, keeping them straight.
- Lower your legs towards the ground with control, then lift them back up towards your chest.
- Engage your core throughout the movement to stabilize your body.
- Aim for 10-12 repetitions.

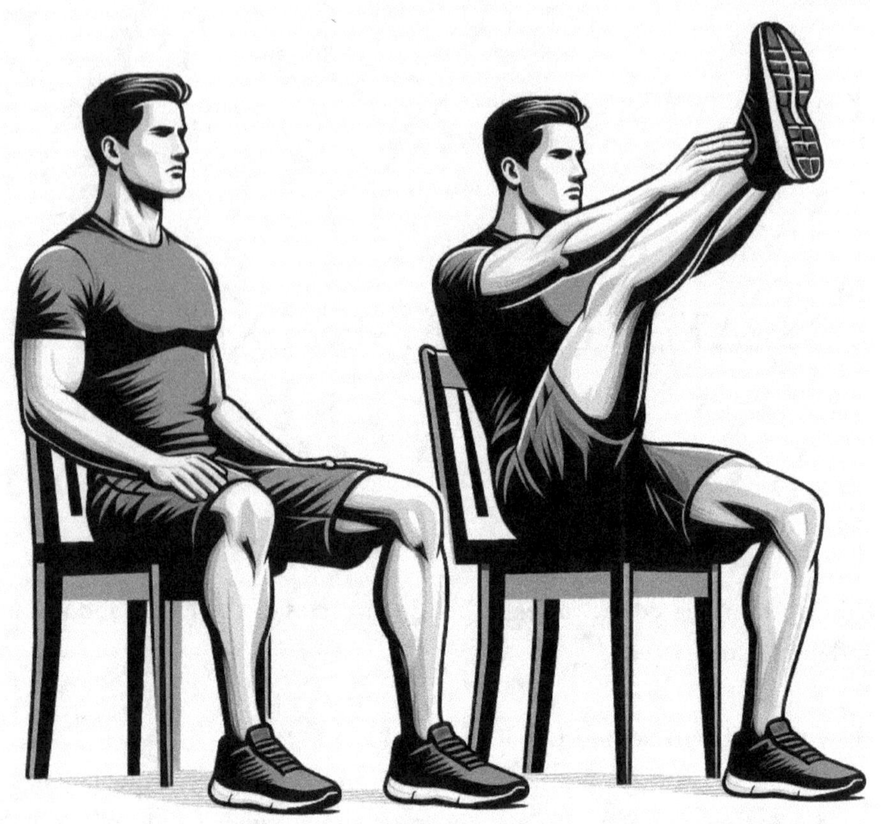

Benefits of Seated Leg Raises:

1. Strengthens lower abdominal muscles.
2. Targets hip flexors.
3. Improves core stability and control.
4. Can be done anywhere with a chair or bench.

29

STANDING BICEP CURLS EXERCISE

28) Standing Bicep Curls:

Description: Standing bicep curls target the muscles of the biceps and forearms.

How to Perform Standing Bicep Curls:

- Stand with your feet hip-width apart and hold a dumbbell in each hand, palms facing forward.
- Keep your elbows close to your sides and curl the weights towards your shoulders, contracting your biceps.
- Lower the weights back down with control, fully extending your arms.
- Repeat for the desired number of repetitions.
- Aim for 10-12 repetitions.

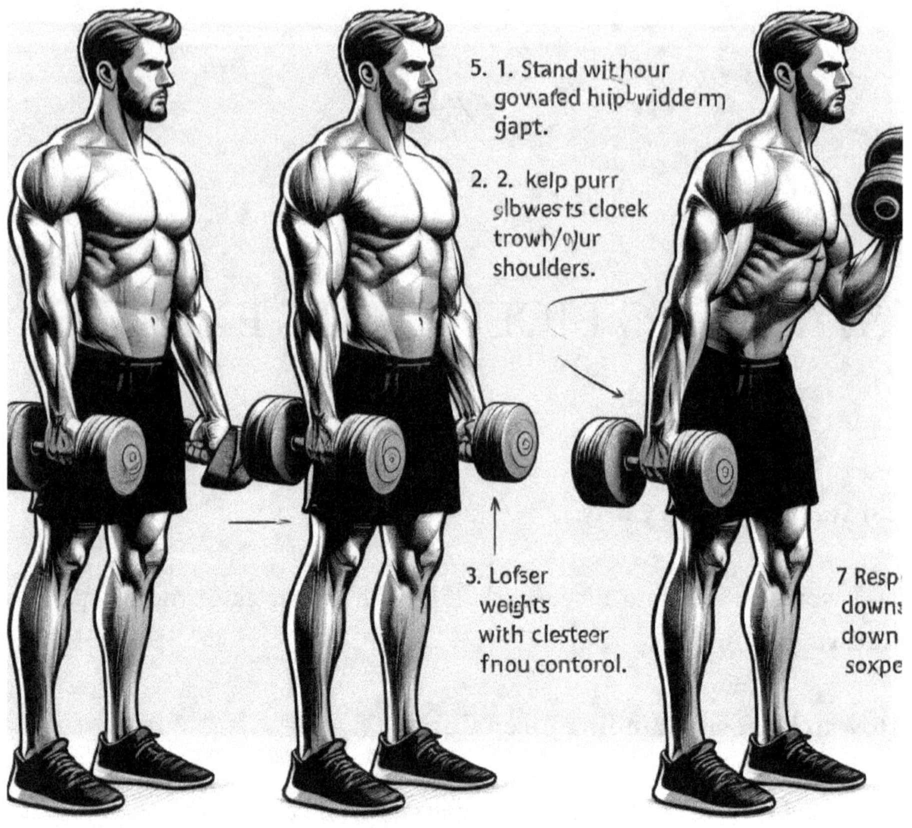

Benefits of Standing Bicep Curls:

1. Strengthens bicep muscles.
2. Improves arm strength and tone.
3. Enhances grip strength and forearm muscles.
4. Can be performed with dumbbells or resistance bands.

30

ORDINARY GLUTE BRIDGE EXERCISE

29) Glute Bridge:

Description: The glute bridge is a lower body exercise that primarily targets the glutes, hamstrings, and lower back.

How to Perform Ordinary Glute Bridge:

- Lie on your back with your knees bent and your feet flat on the ground, hip-width apart.
- Engage your core and squeeze your glutes as you lift your hips towards the ceiling, forming a straight line from your shoulders to your knees.
- Hold the top position for a few seconds, then lower your hips back down to the ground with control.
- Aim for 10-12 repetitions.

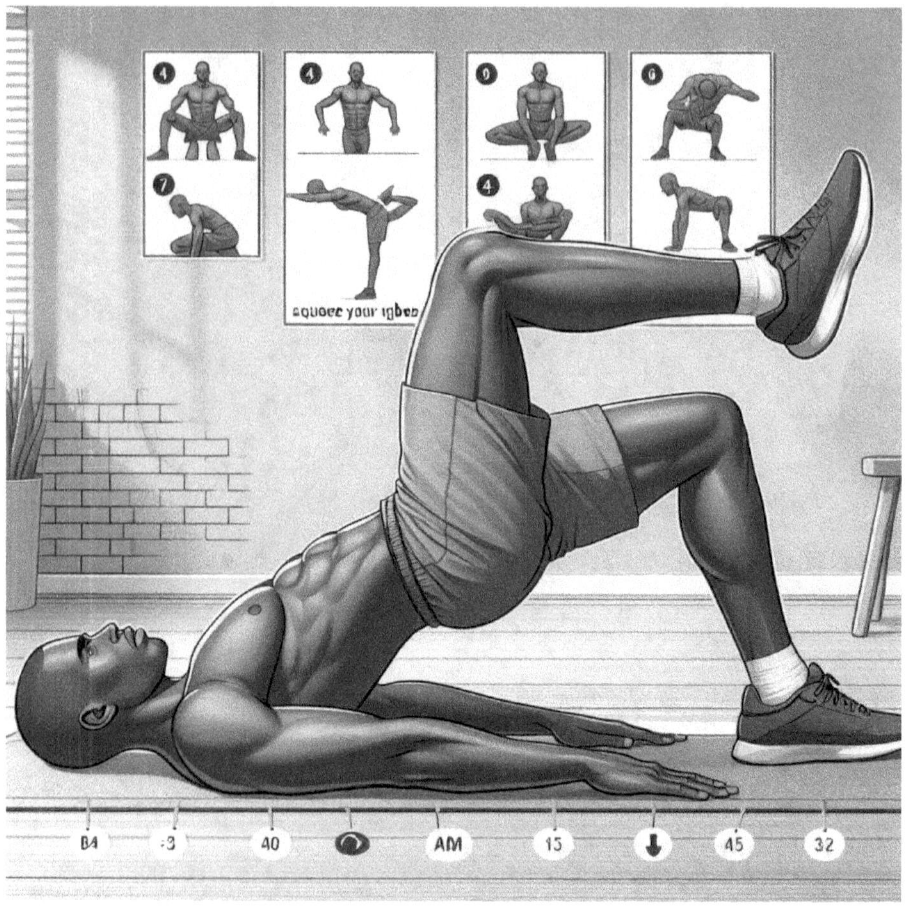

Benefits of Ordinary Glute Bridge:

1. Strengthens glute muscles.
2. Improves hip mobility and stability.
3. Targets hamstrings and lower back muscles.
4. Can help alleviate lower back pain.

31

DUMBBELL ROWS EXERCISE

30) Dumbbell Rows:

Description: Dumbbell rows are a compound exercise that targets the muscles of the upper back, which includes the lats and rhomboids.

How to Perform of Dumbbell Rows:

- Stand with your feet hip-width apart, holding a dumbbell in each hand with your palms facing your body.
- Hinge forward at the hips, keeping your back flat and your core engaged.
- Pull the dumbbells towards your ribcage, squeezing your shoulder blades together at the top of the movement.
- Lower the dumbbells back down with control, fully extending your arms.
- Aim for 10-12 repetitions on each side.

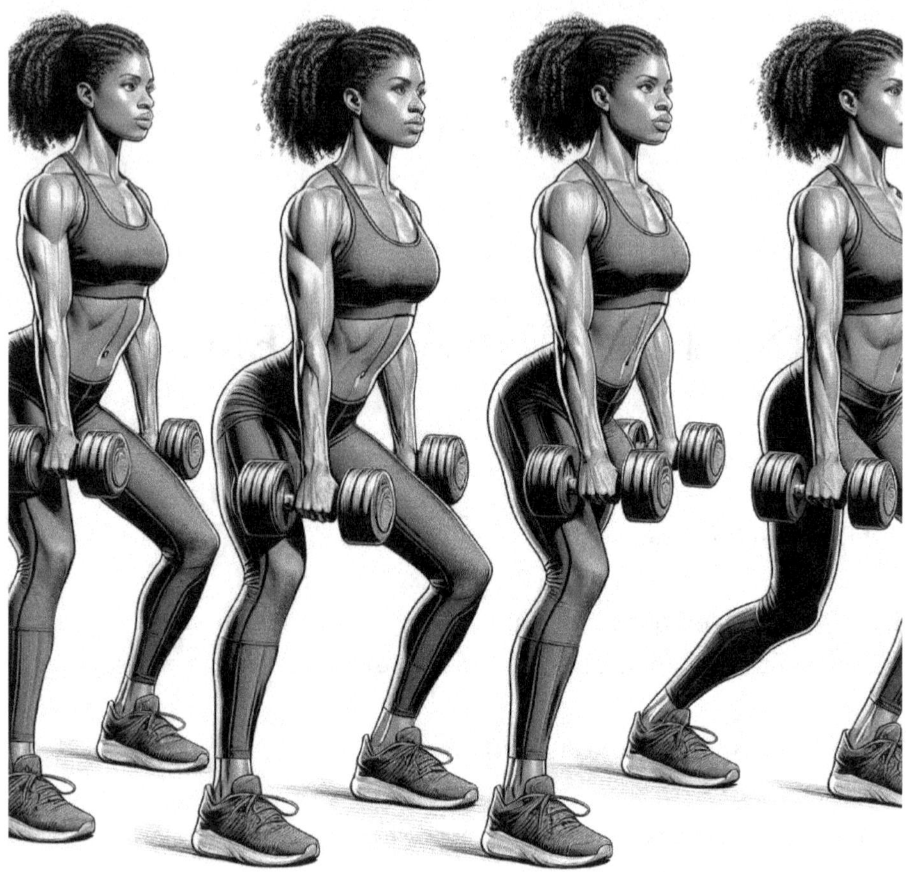

Benefits of Dumbbell Rows:

1. Strengthens upper back muscles.
2. Improves posture and spinal alignment.
3. Targets rear deltoids and bicep muscles.
4. Can help prevent shoulder injuries.

32

BOX JUMPS EXERCISE

31) Box Jumps:

Description: Box jumps are known as plyometric exercises (exercises that go with speed and force of different movements to build muscle power) that target the muscles of the lower body and improve explosive power.

How to Perform Box Jumps:

- Stand in front of a sturdy box or platform with your feet hip-width apart.
- Bend your knees and swing your arms back as you prepare to jump.
- Explosively jump onto the box, landing softly with both feet.
- Stand up tall on top of the box, then step or jump back down to the starting position.
- Aim for 8-10 repetitions.

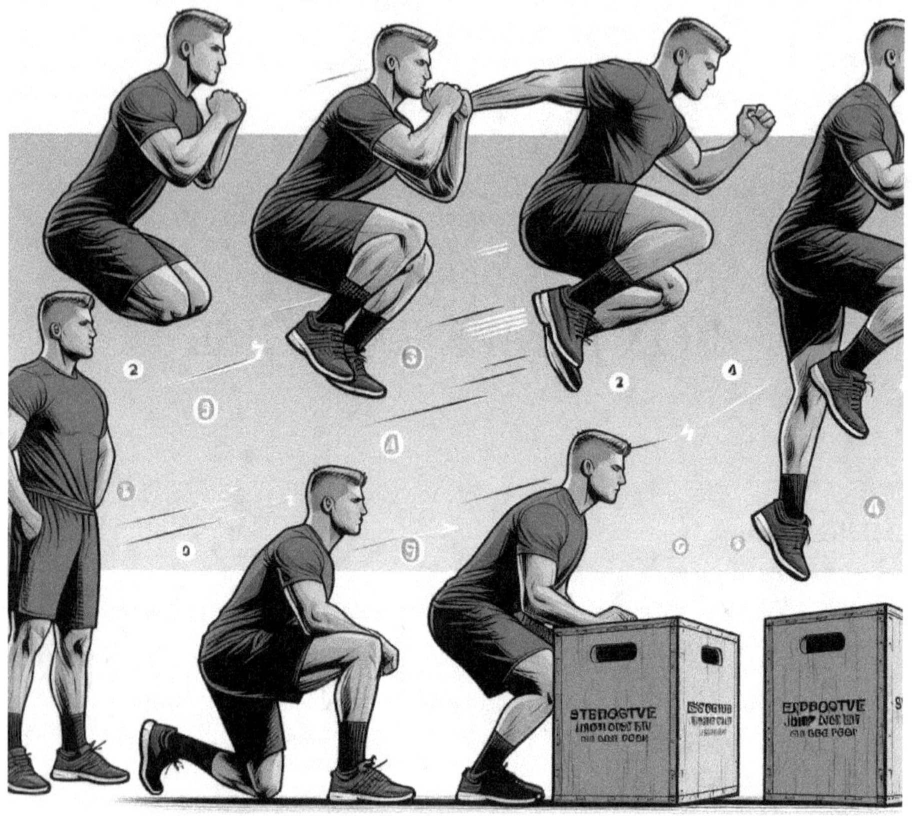

Benefits of Box Jumps:

1. Improves lower body power and explosiveness.
2. Strengthens leg muscles, including quadriceps and calves.
3. Increases cardiovascular fitness.
4. Enhances coordination and agility.

33

SEATED HAMSTRING CURLS EXERCISE

32) Seated Hamstring Curls:

Description: Hamstring curls target the muscles of the hamstrings, helping to strengthen and tone the back of the thighs.

How to Perform Seated Hamstring Curls:

- Sit on the hamstring curl machine with your back against the pad and your legs extended in front of you.
- Adjust the machine's settings so that the pad rests just above your ankles.
- Grasp the handles for stability and keep your torso upright.
- Exhale and curl your legs upward by flexing your knees until your hamstrings are fully contracted.
- Hold the peak contraction briefly, then inhale and slowly lower the weight back to the starting position.
- Repeat for the desired number of repetitions.

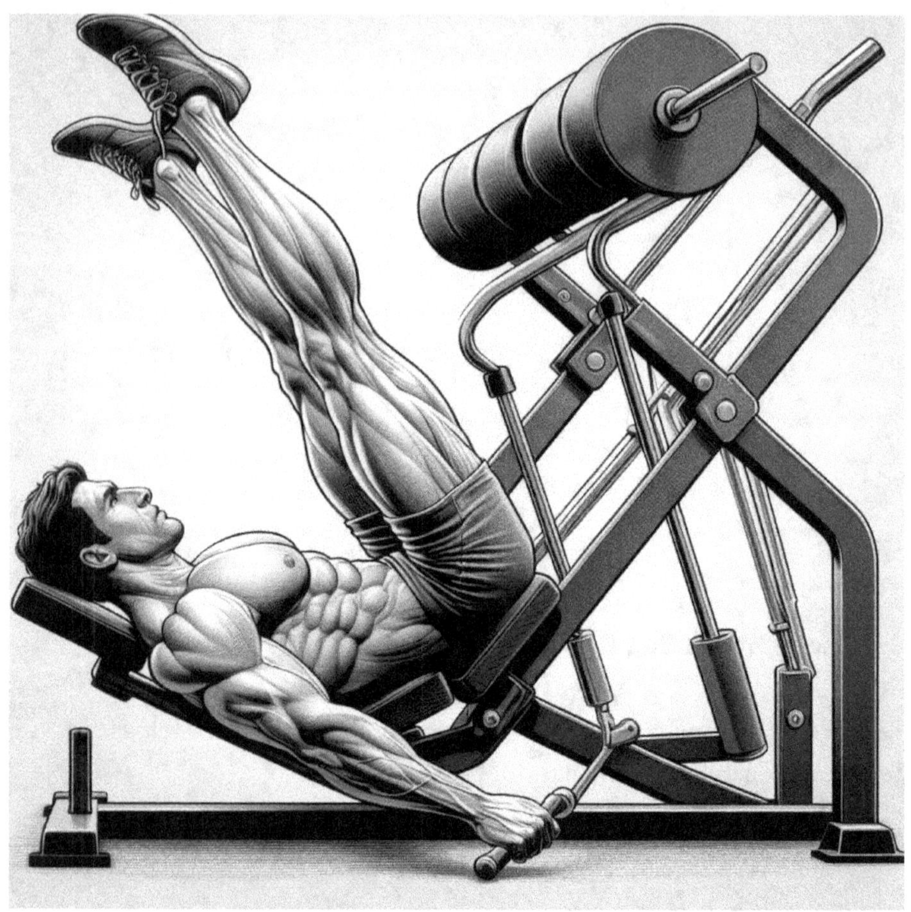

Benefits of Seated Hamstring Curls:

1. Strengthens hamstring muscles.
2. Improves knee stability and function.
3. Helps prevent hamstring injuries.
4. Can be performed using a leg curl machine or resistance bands.

34

CALF RAISES EXERCISE

33) Calf Raises:

Description: Calf raises target the muscles of the calves, including the gastrocnemius and soleus.

How to Perform Calf Raises:

- Stand with your feet hip-width apart and your hands resting on a stable surface for support.
- Rise up onto the balls of your feet as high as possible, lifting your heels off the ground.
- Hold the top position for a moment, then lower your heels back down to the starting position with control.
- Aim for 15-20 repetitions.

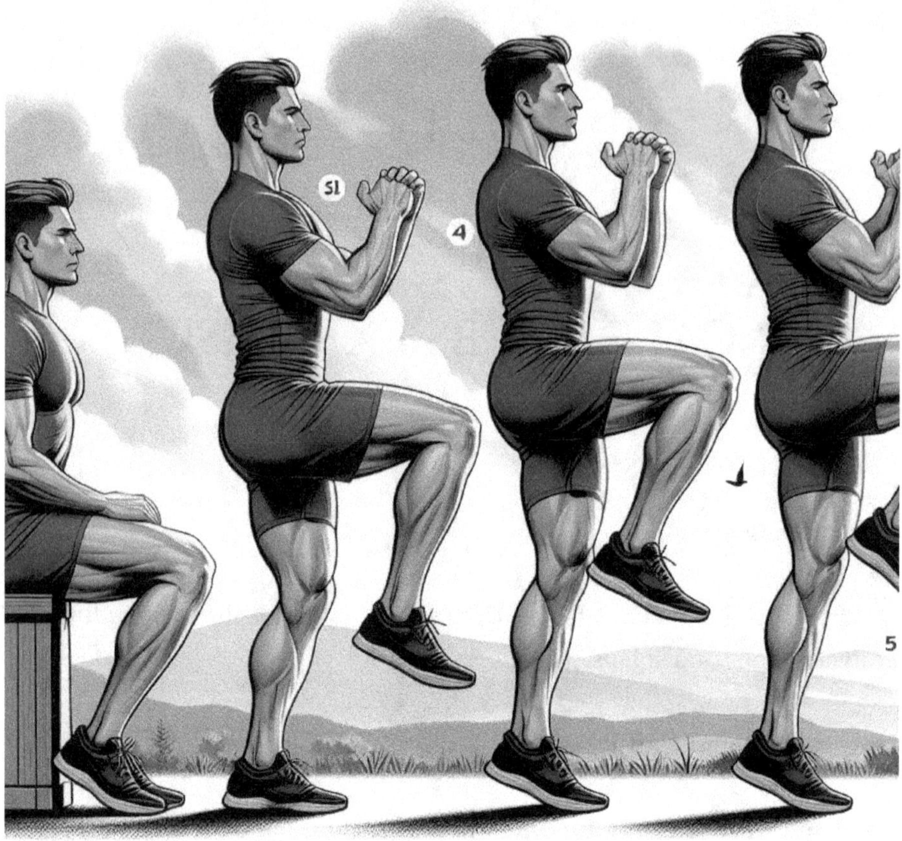

Benefits of Calf Raises:

1. Strengthens calf muscles.
2. Improves ankle stability and balance.
3. Enhances lower body strength and power.
4. Can be performed anywhere with minimal equipment.

35

TRICEP PUSHDOWNS EXERCISE

34) Tricep Pushdowns:

Description: Tricep pushdowns target the triceps, the muscles on the back of your upper arms.

How to Perform Tricep Pushdowns:

- Stand facing a cable machine with a high pulley attachment.
- Grab the bar or rope attachment with an overhand grip, hands shoulder-width apart.
- Keep your elbows close to your sides and your upper arms stationary as you push the bar or rope down until your arms are fully extended.
- Slowly return to the starting position with control.
- Aim for 10-12 repetitions.

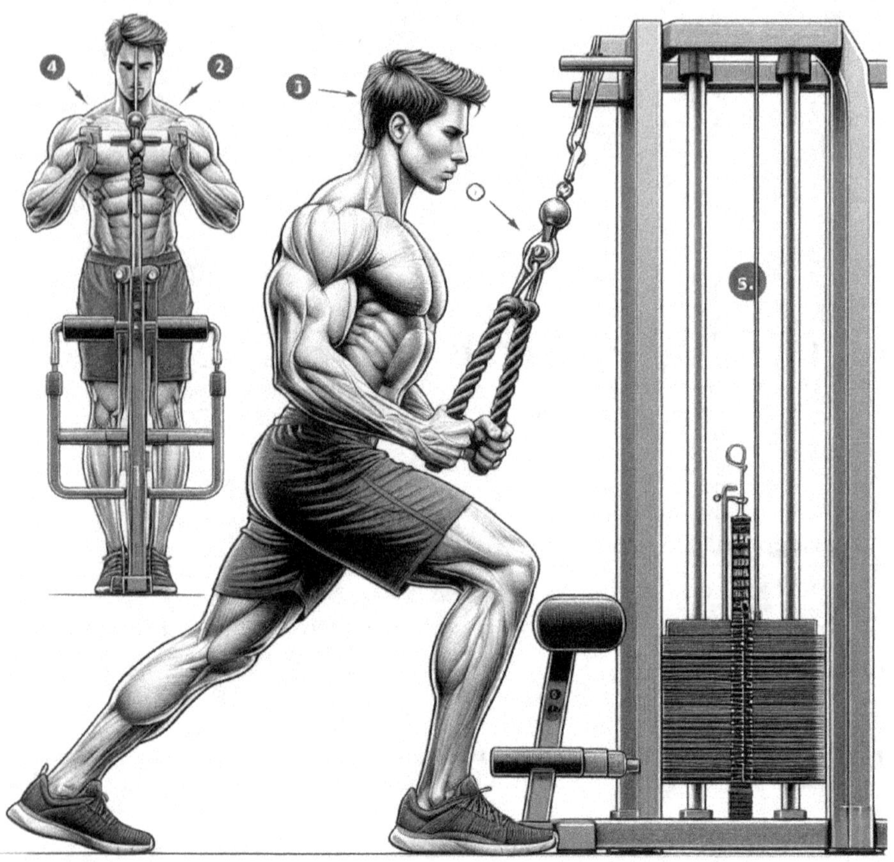

Benefits of Tricep Pushdowns:

1. Strengthens tricep muscles.
2. Helps tone and define the back of the arms.
3. Can be performed with different attachments for variation.

36

WALL PUSH-UPS EXERCISE

35) Wall Push-Ups:

Description: Wall push-ups are a beginner-friendly variation of the traditional push-up exercise, targeting the chest, shoulders, and arms.

How to Perform Wall Push-Ups:

- Stand facing a wall with your feet hip-width apart.
- Place your hands on the wall slightly wider than shoulder-width apart, at shoulder height.
- Lean forward and bend your elbows to lower your chest towards the wall.
- Push through your palms to straighten your arms and return to the starting position.
- Aim for 10-12 repetitions.

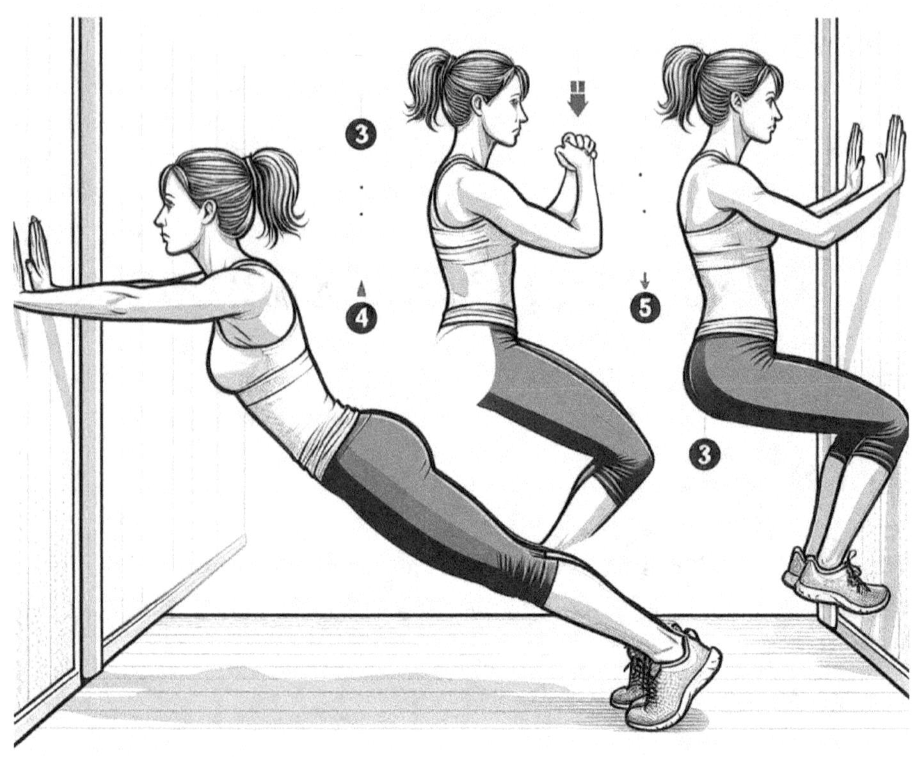

Benefits of Wall Push-Ups:

1. Strengthens upper body muscles.
2. Provides a less intense variation of push-ups for beginners.
3. Improves chest and shoulder strength.

37

LATERAL BAND WALKS EXERCISE

36) Lateral Band Walks:

Description: Lateral band walks target the muscles of the hips, including the glutes and abductors.

How to Perform Wall Push-Ups:

- Place a resistance band around your legs, just above your knees.
- Stand with your feet hip-width apart and your knees slightly bent.
- Take a step to the side with one foot, then follow with the other foot, maintaining tension on the band.
- Continue stepping sideways for a few steps, then reverse direction and return to the starting position.
- Aim for 10-12 steps in each direction.

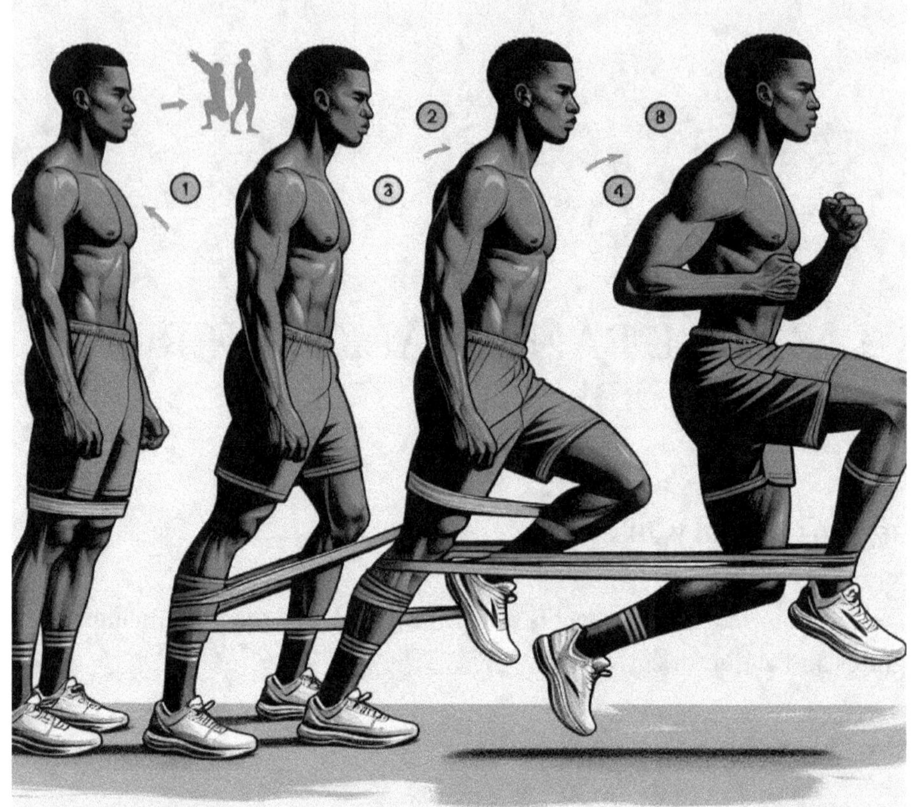

Benefits of Wall Push-Ups:

1. Strengthens hip abductor muscles.
2. Improves hip stability and balance.
3. Helps prevent knee injuries by strengthening the muscles around the
   knee joint.

38

REVERSE FLYES EXERCISE

37) Reverse Flyes:

Description: Reverse flyes target the muscles of the upper back, including the rear deltoids and rhomboids.

How to Perform Reverse Flyes:

- Stand with your feet hip-width apart and hold a pair of dumbbells in front of your thighs, palms facing each other.
- Hinge forward at the hips, keeping your back flat and your core engaged.
- Lift the dumbbells out to the sides, squeezing your shoulder blades together at the top of the movement.
- Slowly lower the dumbbells back down with control.
- Aim for 10-12 repetitions.

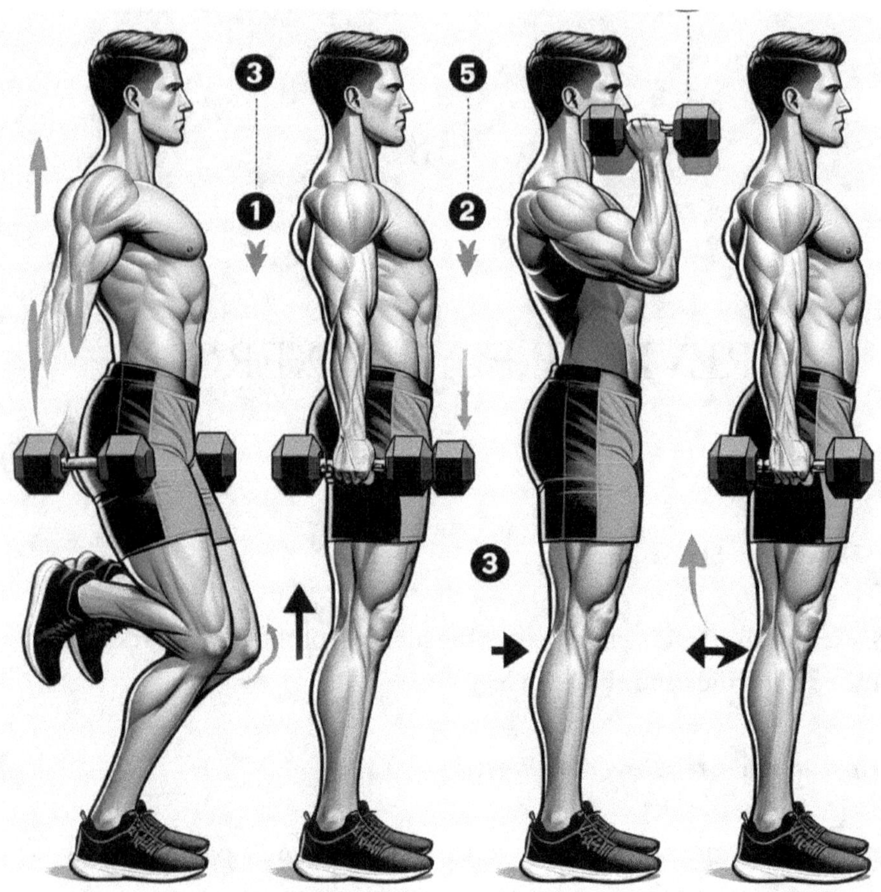

Benefits of Reverse Flyes:

1. Strengthens upper back muscles.
2. Improves posture by targeting the muscles that help retract the shoulders.
3. Can help prevent shoulder injuries by strengthening the muscles around the shoulder joint.

39

STEP-UPS EXERCISE

38) Step-Ups:

Description: Step-ups are a lower body exercise that targets the quadriceps, hamstrings, and glutes.

How to Perform of Step-Ups:

- Stand in front of a sturdy bench or platform.
- Step up onto the bench with one foot, driving through your heel to lift your body up.
- Fully extend your hip and knee at the top of the movement, then step back down with control.
- Repeat on the same leg for a set number of repetitions, then switch legs.
- Aim for 10-12 repetitions on each leg.

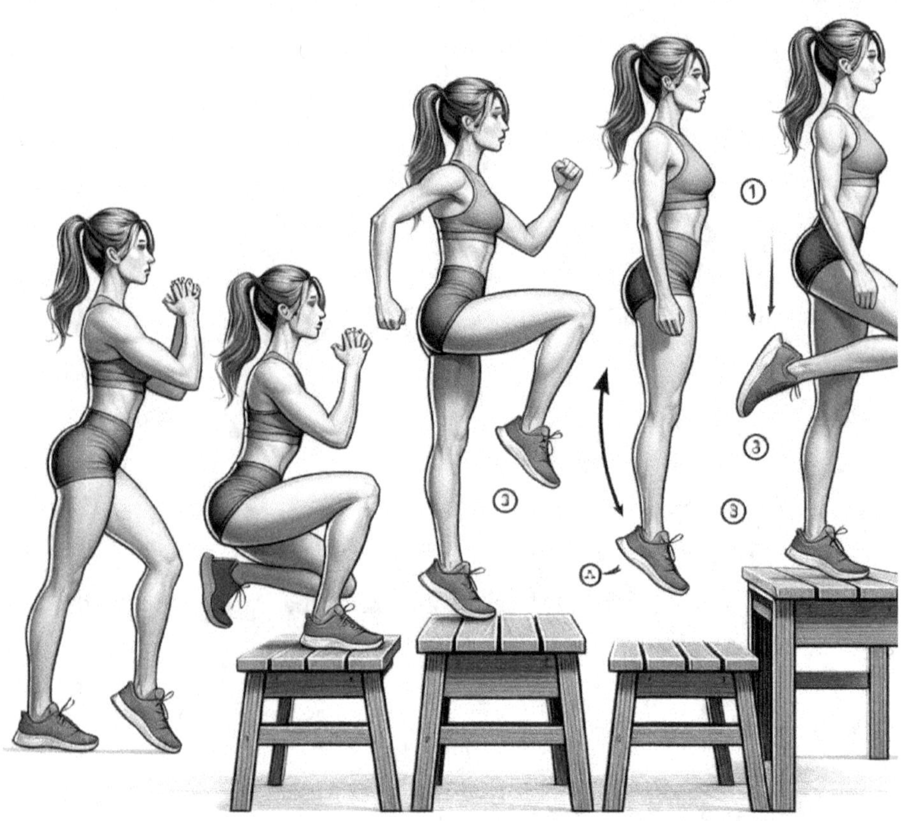

Benefits of Step-Ups:

1. Strengthens lower body muscles.
2. Improves balance and stability.
3. Provides a functional movement pattern similar to climbing stairs.

40

CROSS-BODY BICYCLE CRUNCHES EXERCISE

39) Cross-Body Bicycle Crunches:

Description: Cross-body bicycle crunches are a variation of the traditional bicycle crunch exercise. Instead of bringing your elbows towards the opposite knee as in the traditional version, you twist your torso to bring your right elbow towards your left knee, and vice versa. This twisting motion engages your oblique muscles more intensely, helping to strengthen and tone your sides.

How to Perform Cross-Body Bicycle Crunches:

- Start by lying on your back with your knees bent and feet flat on the floor.
- Place your hands behind your head, elbows pointing out to the sides.
- Lift your shoulder blades off the ground, engaging your core muscles.
- Extend your right leg out straight while simultaneously twisting your torso to bring your right elbow towards your left knee.
- Focus on bringing your elbow and knee as close together as possible while keeping your shoulder blades off the ground.

- Return to the starting position and repeat the motion on the other side, bringing your left elbow towards your right knee.
- Continue alternating sides in a controlled manner, maintaining a steady pace.
- Aim for 10-12 repetitions on each side.

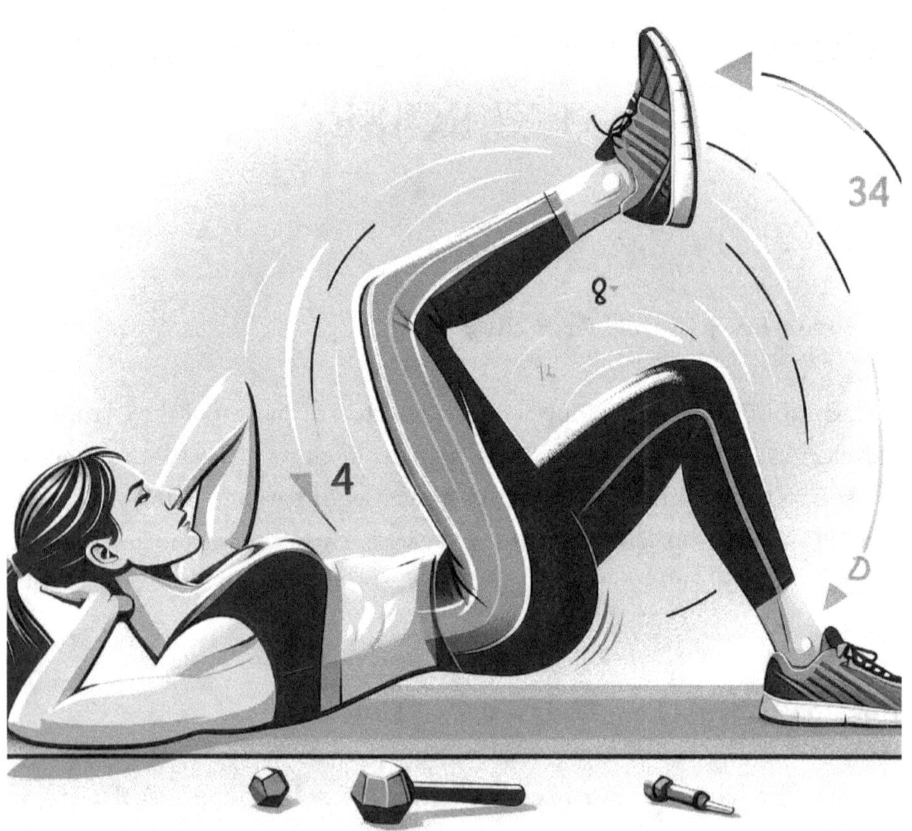

Benefits of Cross-Body Bicycle Crunches:

1. Engages Obliques: The twisting motion targets the oblique muscles on the sides of your abdomen, helping to strengthen and define your

waistline.

2. Improves Core Stability: By lifting your shoulder blades off the ground and engaging your core muscles, cross-body bicycle crunches help improve core stability and balance.

3. Enhances Coordination: Coordinating the twisting motion with the leg movement challenges your coordination and motor skills.

4. Increases Intensity: Compared to traditional bicycle crunches, the cross-body variation increases the intensity of the exercise, making it more challenging and effective for building abdominal strength and endurance.

41

PLANK SHOULDER TAPS EXERCISE

40) Plank Shoulder Taps:

Description: Plank shoulder taps add an extra challenge to the traditional plank exercise by incorporating movement of the arms, shoulders, and core.

How to Perform Plank Shoulder Taps:

- Start in a forearm plank position with your elbows directly under your shoulders and your body forming a straight line from head to heels.
- Keeping your hips stable and core engaged, lift one hand off the ground and tap the opposite shoulder.
- Return to the starting position and repeat on the other side.
- Continue alternating sides while maintaining proper plank form.
- Aim for 10-12 taps on each shoulder.

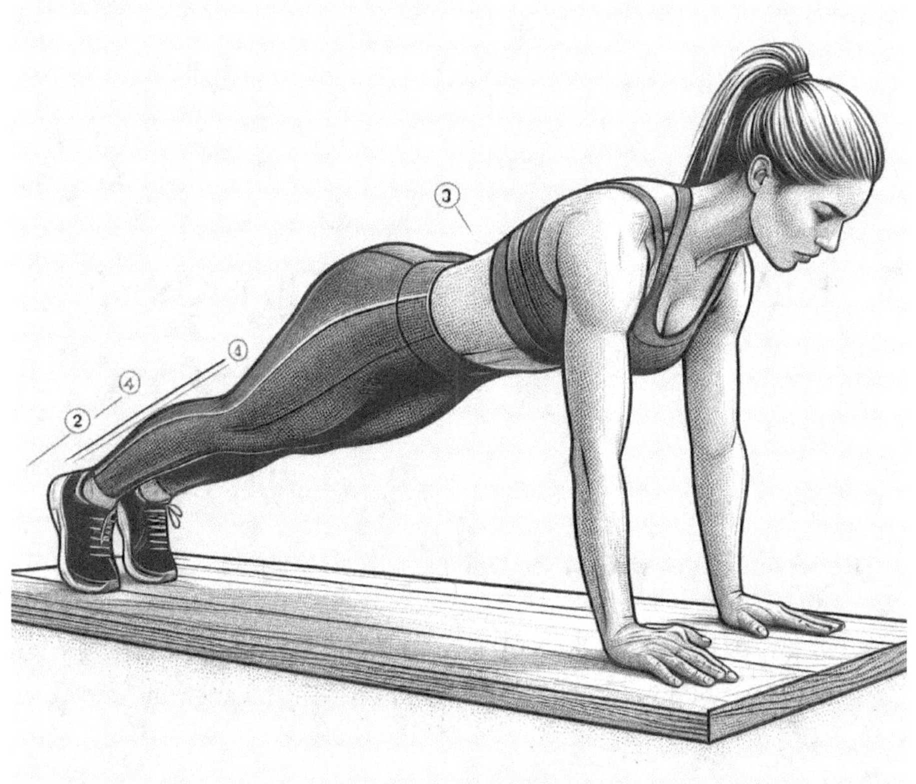

Benefits of Plank Shoulder Taps:

1. Increases core stability and strength.
2. Targets shoulder stabilizer muscles.
3. Improves coordination and proprioception.

42

REVERSE LUNGES WITH KNEE DRIVE EXERCISE

41) Reverse Lunges with Knee Drive:

Description: Reverse lunges with knee drive target the quadriceps, hamstrings, glutes, and hip flexors, while also improving balance and coordination.

How to Perform Reverse Lunges with Knee Drive:

- Stand with your feet hip-width apart and your hands on your hips.
- Step back with your right foot into a reverse lunge, bending both knees to lower your body towards the ground.
- Push through your left heel to return to the starting position, driving your right knee up towards your chest.
- Lower your right foot back to the ground and repeat on the other side.
- Aim for 10-12 repetitions on each leg.

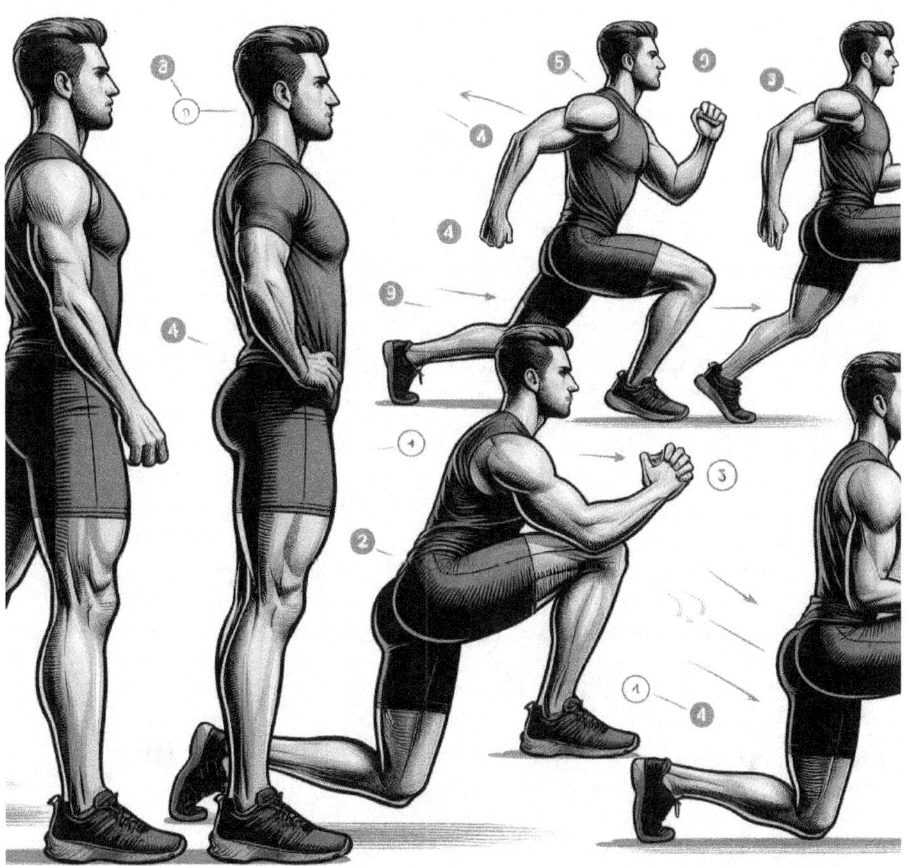

Benefits of Reverse Lunges with Knee Drive:

1. Strengthens lower body muscles.
2. Improves balance and stability.
3. Engages core muscles for stabilization.

43

INCHWORMS EXERCISE

42) Inchworms:

Description: Inchworms are a full-body exercise that targets the core, shoulders, hamstrings, and calves.

How to Perform Inchworms:

- Stand with your feet hip-width apart and hinge forward at the hips to place your hands on the ground.
- Walk your hands forward until you reach a high plank position, keeping your core engaged and your body forming a straight line from head to heels.
- Pause briefly in the plank position, then walk your hands back towards your feet, keeping your legs as straight as possible.
- Stand up tall and repeat for the desired number of repetitions.
- Aim for 8-10 repetitions.

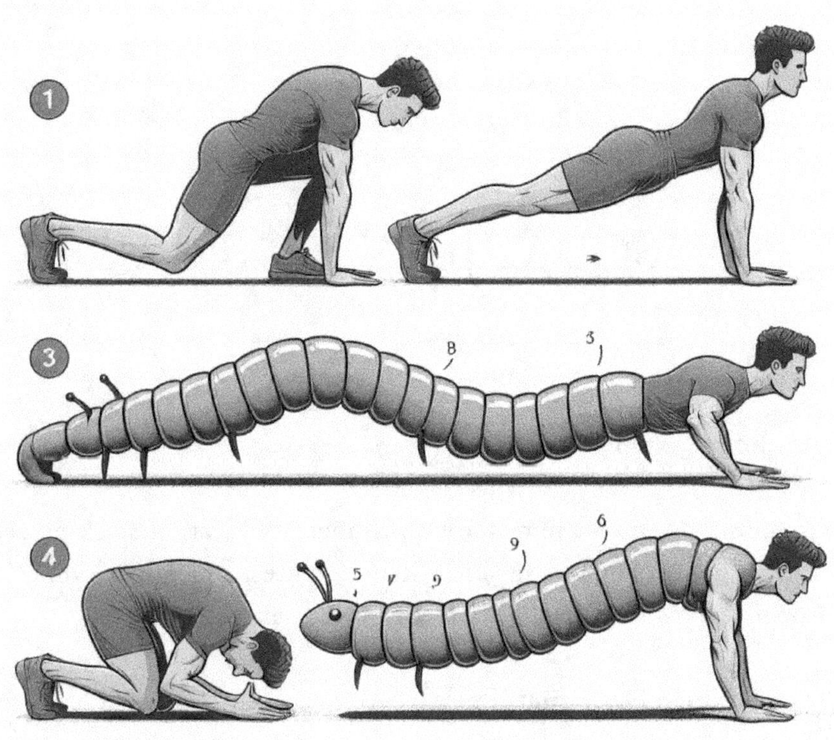

Benefits of Inchworms:

1. Strengthens core muscles.
2. Improves shoulder stability and strength.
3. Increases flexibility in the hamstrings and calves.

44

BOX SQUAT JUMPS EXERCISE

43) Box Squat Jumps:

Description: Box squat jumps are a plyometric exercise (check exercise 30) that targets the quadriceps, hamstrings, glutes, and calves, while also improving explosive power and athletic performance.

How to Perform Box Squat Jumps:

- Stand facing a sturdy box or platform with your feet hip-width apart.
- Lower into a squat position, then explosively jump onto the box, landing softly with both feet.
- Step or jump back down to the starting position and immediately lower into another squat to prepare for the next jump.
- Aim for 8-10 repetitions.

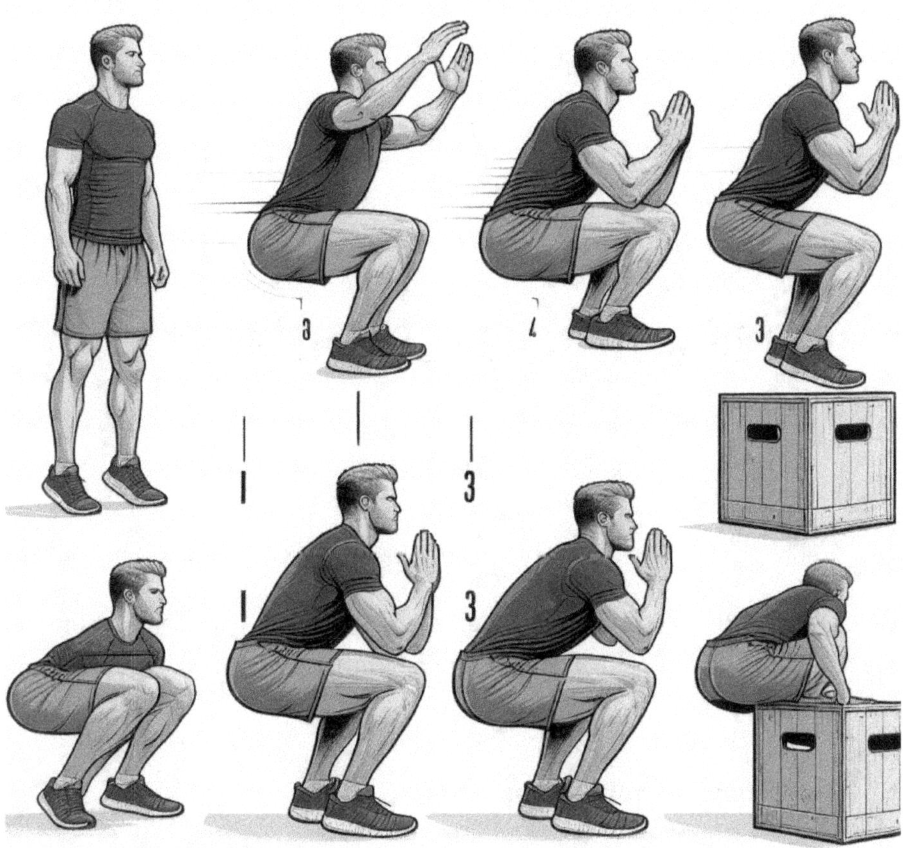

Benefits of Box Squat Jumps:

1. Improves lower body power and explosiveness.
2. Strengthens leg muscles.
3. Enhances athletic performance.

45

PISTOL SQUATS EXERCISE

44) Pistol Squats:

Description: Pistol squats are a challenging single-leg exercise that targets the quadriceps, hamstrings, glutes, and core muscles, while also improving balance and stability.

How to Perform Pistol Squats:

- Stand on one leg with your other leg extended straight out in front of you.
- Lower your body down into a squat position, keeping your chest up and your back straight.
- Keep your extended leg off the ground throughout the movement.
- Push through your heel to return to the starting position.
- Aim for 5-8 repetitions on each leg.

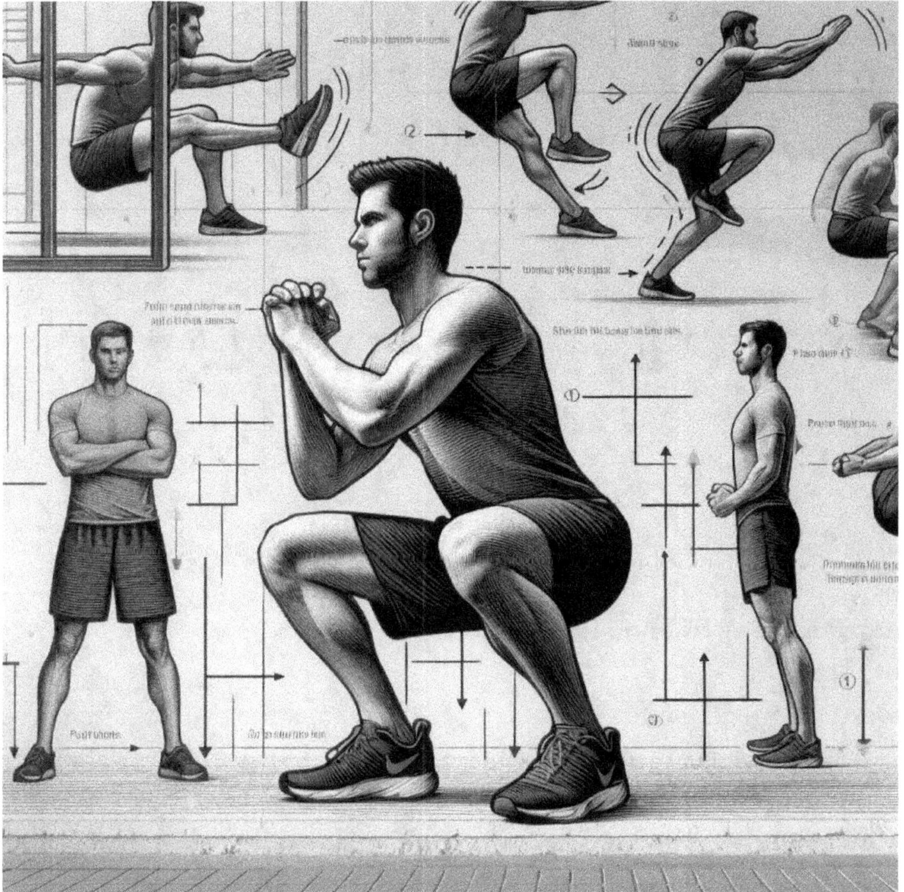

Benefits of Pistol Squats:

1. Strengthens lower body muscles.
2. Improves balance and stability.
3. Challenges core muscles.

46

SINGLE-LEG ROMANIAN DEADLIFTS EXERCISE

45) Single-Leg Romanian Deadlifts:

Description: Single-leg Romanian deadlifts target the hamstrings, glutes, lower back, and core muscles, while also improving balance and stability.

How to Perform Single-Leg Romanian Deadlifts:

- Stand on one leg with a slight bend in the knee and hold a dumbbell or kettlebell in one hand.
- Hinge forward at the hips, keeping your back flat and your free leg extended straight behind you for balance.
- Lower the weight towards the ground while simultaneously lifting your back leg until your body forms a straight line from head to heel.
- Pause briefly at the bottom, then return to the starting position by driving through your standing heel and squeezing your glutes.
- Aim for 8-10 repetitions on each leg.

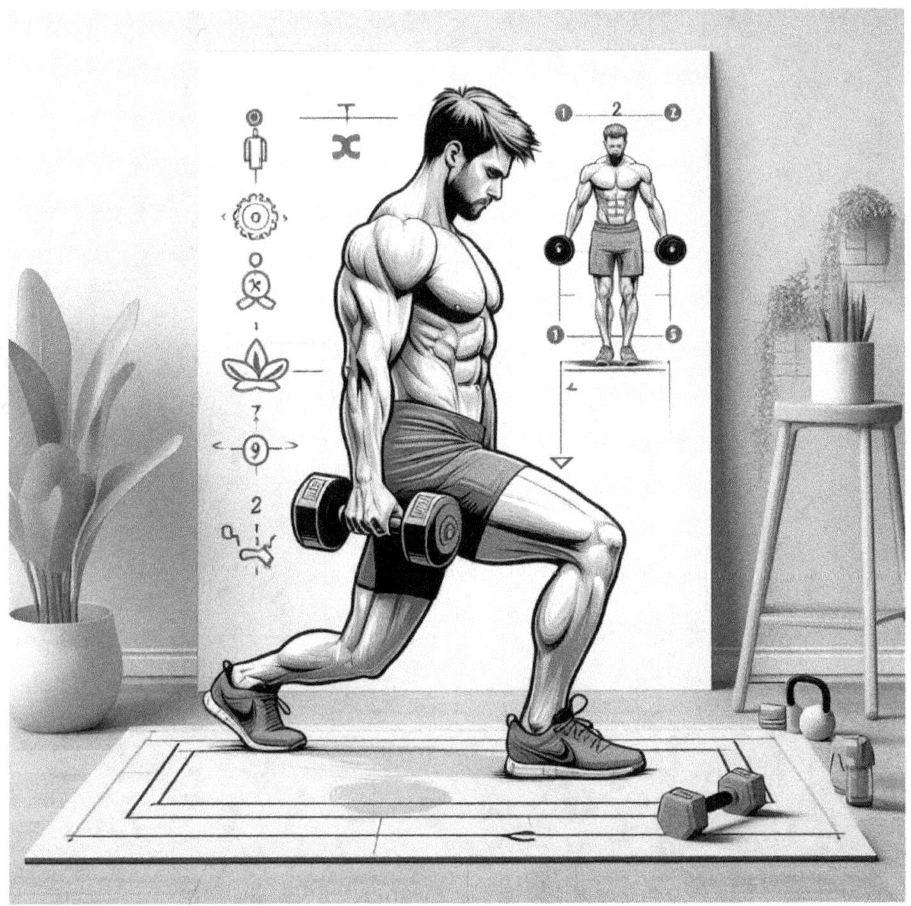

Benefits of Single-Leg Romanian Deadlifts:

1. Strengthens posterior chain muscles.
2. Improves balance and stability.
3. Challenges core muscles.

47

KETTLEBELL SWINGS EXERCISE

46) Kettlebell Swings:

Description: Kettlebell swings are a dynamic exercise that targets the hamstrings, glutes, lower back, and shoulders, while also providing cardiovascular benefits.

How to Perform Kettlebell Swings:

- Stand with your feet slightly wider than hip-width apart and hold a kettlebell with both hands in front of you.
- Hinge at the hips and lower the kettlebell between your legs, keeping your back flat and your chest up.
- Drive through your heels to swing the kettlebell up to shoulder height, using the momentum from your hips.
- Allow the kettlebell to swing back between your legs, then immediately hinge at the hips to begin the next repetition.
- Aim for 12-15 repetitions.

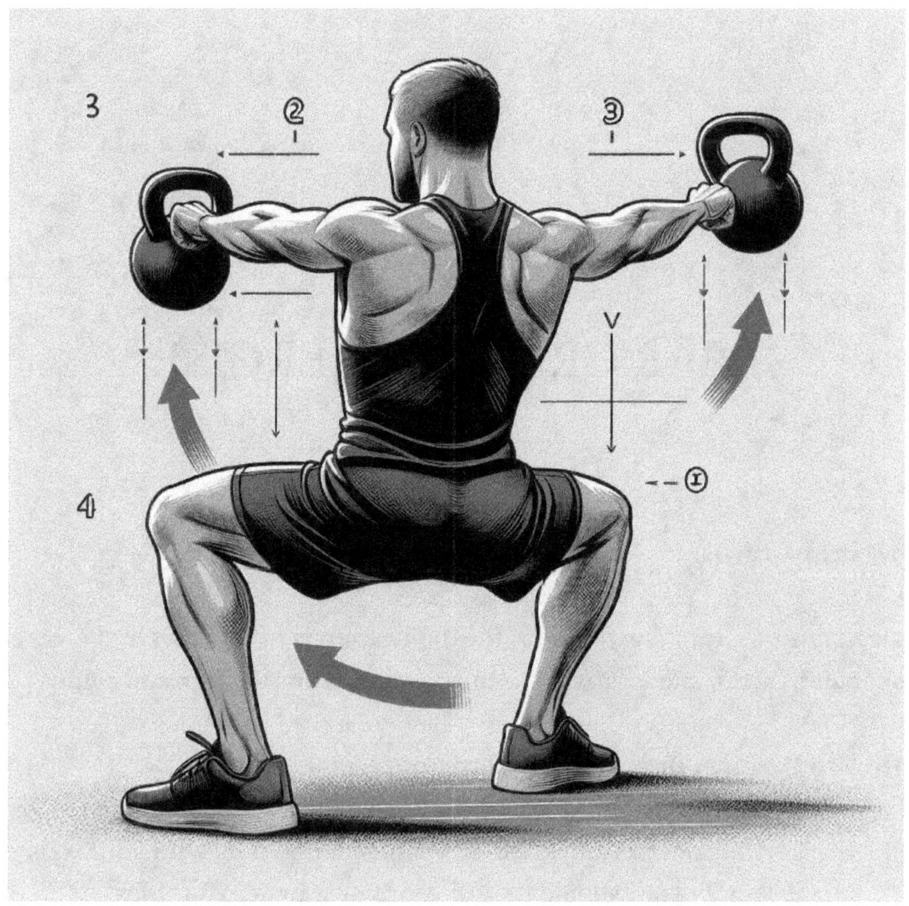

Benefits Kettlebell Swings:

1. Strengthens posterior chain muscles.
2. Improves explosive power and athletic performance.
3. Increases heart rate for cardiovascular benefits.

48

BEAR CRAWLS EXERCISE

47) Bear Crawls:

Description: Bear crawls are a full-body exercise that targets the core, shoulders, arms, and legs, while also improving coordination and agility.

How to Perform Bear Crawls:

- Start on your hands and knees in a tabletop position, with your wrists aligned under your shoulders and your knees under your hips.
- Lift your knees off the ground a few inches, keeping your back flat and your core engaged.
- Crawl forward by moving your opposite hand and foot simultaneously, maintaining a stable core throughout.
- Continue crawling forward for a set distance or time, then reverse direction and crawl backward.
- Aim for 20-30 seconds of crawling.

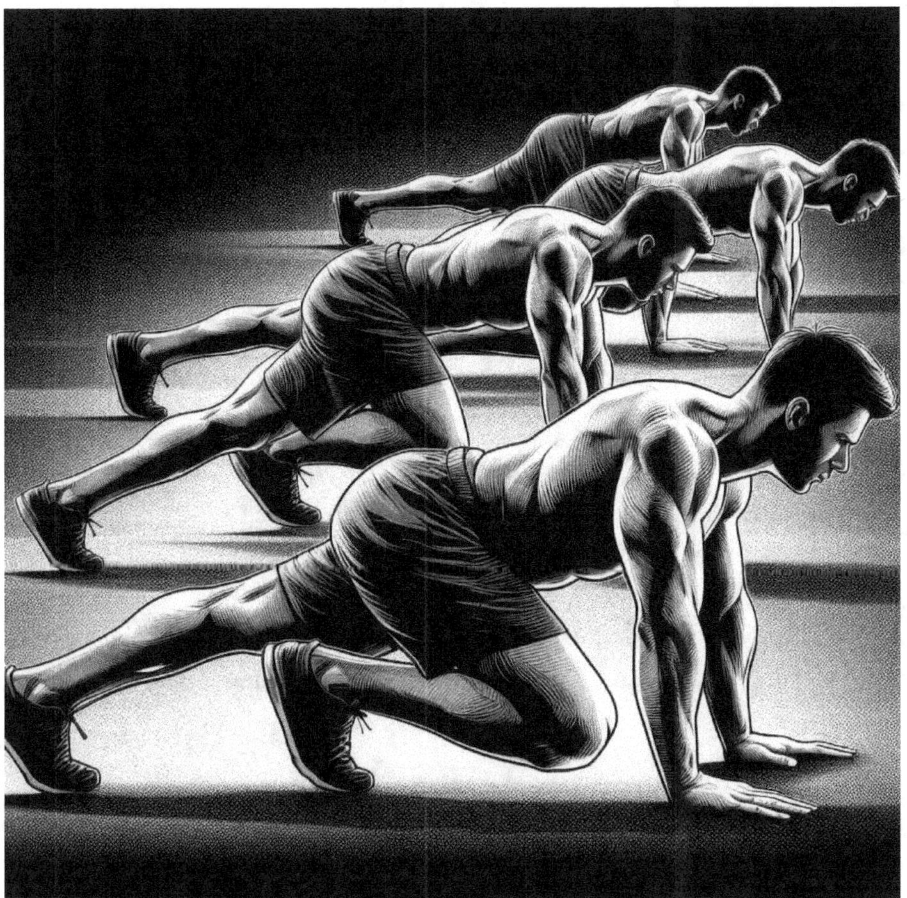

Benefits of Bear Crawls:

1. Strengthens core muscles.
2. Improves shoulder and arm strength.
3. Increases coordination and agility.

49

HOLLOW BODY HOLD EXERCISE

48) Hollow Body Hold:

Description: The hollow body hold is an isometric exercise (when the muscles are contracted without any movement at the surrounding joints) that targets the core muscles, including the abdominals and lower back.

How to Perform Hollow Body Hold:

- Lie on your back with your arms extended overhead and your legs straight out in front of you.
- Lift your shoulders and legs off the ground, keeping your lower back pressed into the floor.
- Engage your core and hold the position for as long as possible, maintaining a straight line from head to heels.
- Keep your arms and legs lifted a few inches off the ground throughout the hold.
- Aim for 30-60 seconds.

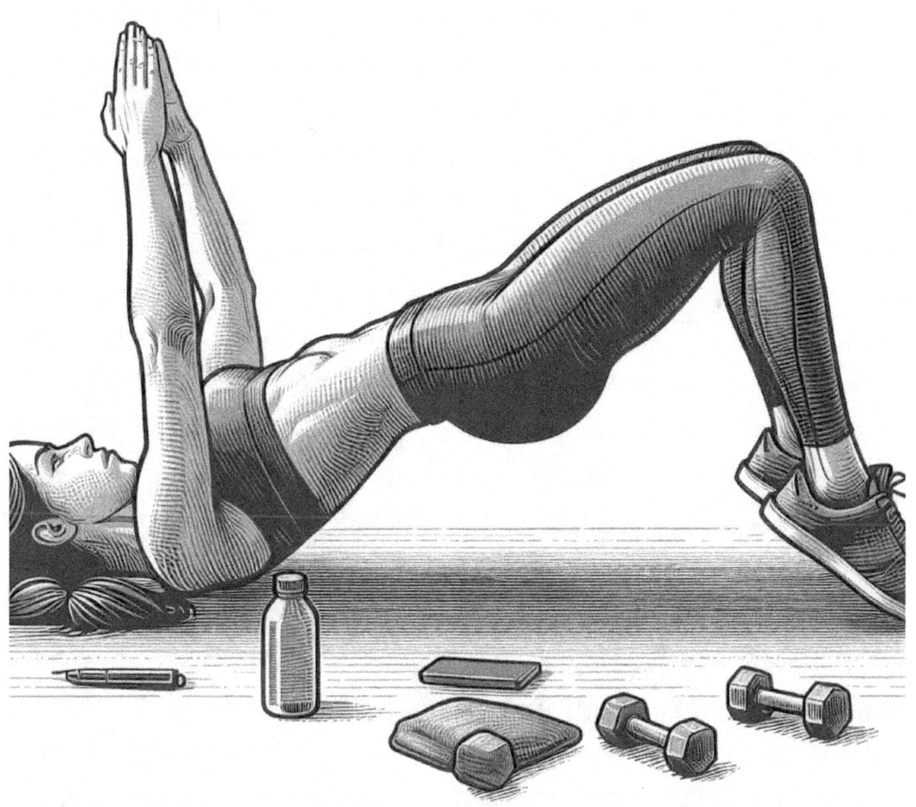

Benefits of Hollow Body Hold:

1. Strengthens core muscles.
2. Improves abdominal endurance.
3. Helps prevent lower back pain.

50

RENEGADE ROWS EXERCISE

49) Renegade Rows:

Description: Renegade rows are a compound exercise that targets the back, shoulders, arms, and core muscles.

How to Perform Renegade Rows:

- Start in a high plank position with a dumbbell in each hand, wrists aligned under shoulders.
- Keeping your core engaged and hips stable, row one dumbbell up towards your hip, retracting your shoulder blade.
- Lower the dumbbell back to the ground and repeat on the opposite side.
- Continue alternating rows while maintaining proper plank form.
- Aim for 10-12 repetitions on each side.

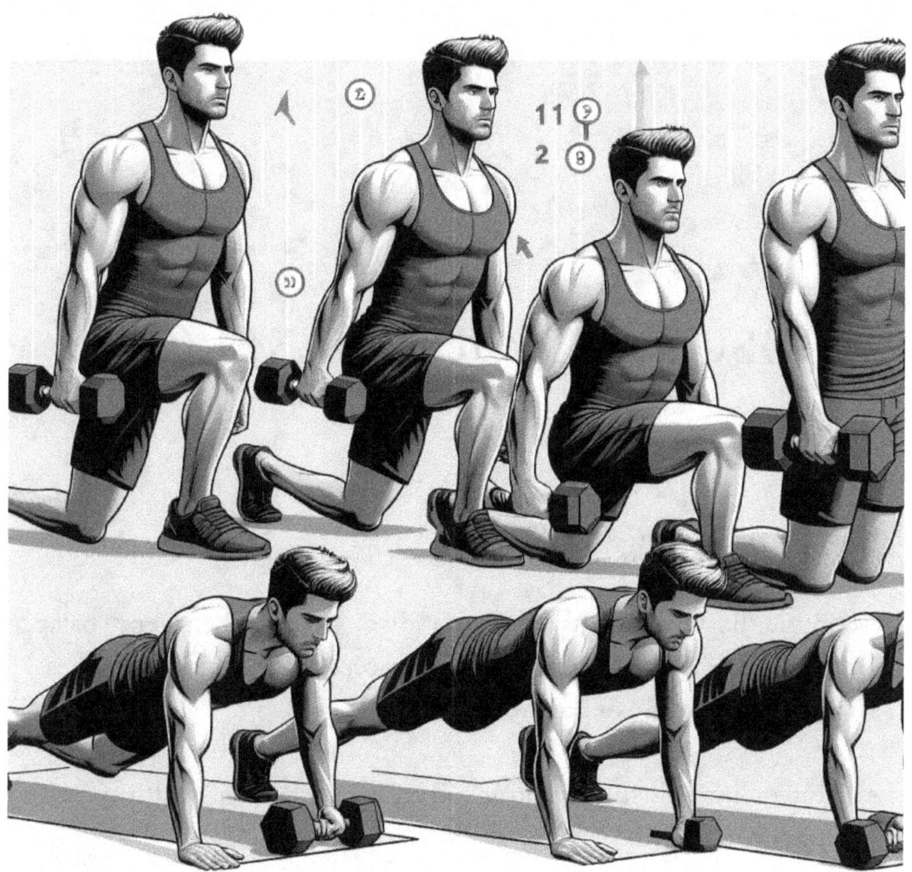

Benefits of Renegade Rows:

1. Strengthens back and shoulder muscles.
2. Engages core muscles for stabilization.
3. Improves grip strength.

51

BOSU BALL SQUATS EXERCISE

50) Bosu Ball Squats:

Description: Bosu ball squats are a variation of squats that challenge balance and stability, while also targeting the quadriceps, hamstrings, and glutes.

How to Perform Bosu Ball Squats:

- Stand on the flat side of a Bosu ball with your feet hip-width apart and your core engaged.
- Lower into a squat by bending your knees and sitting back into your hips, keeping your chest up and your back flat.
- Press through your heels to return to the starting position, squeezing your glutes at the top of the movement.
- Aim for 10-12 repetitions.

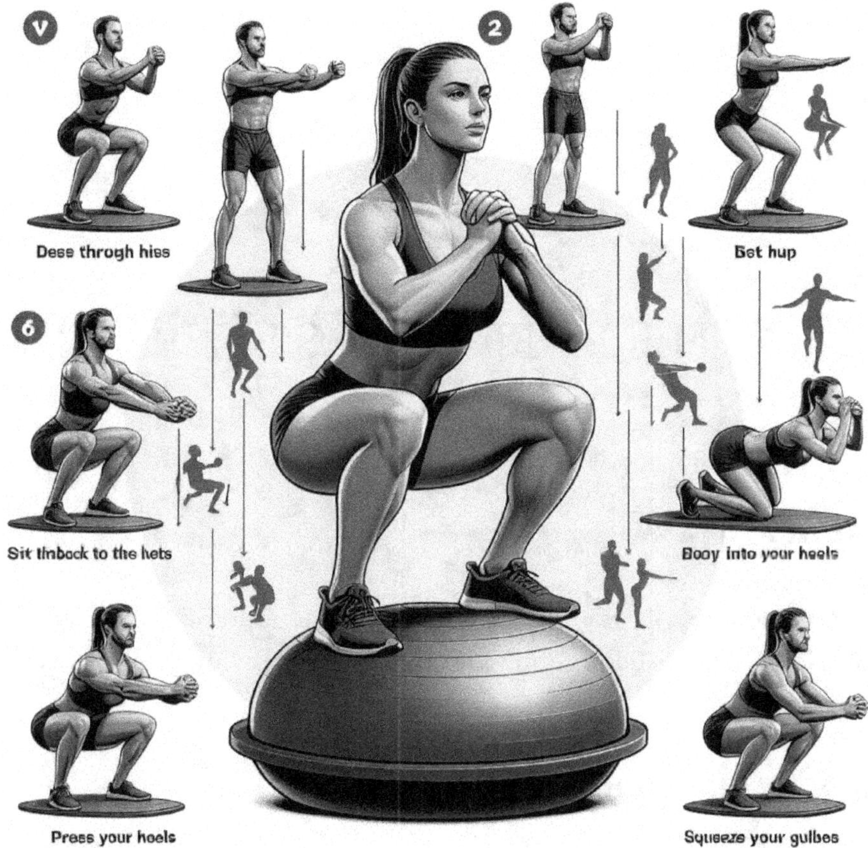

Benefits of Bosu Ball Squats:

1. Strengthens lower body muscles.
2. Improves balance and stability.
3. Engages core muscles for stabilization.

52

BATTLE ROPE WAVES EXERCISE

51) Battle Rope Waves:

Description: Battle rope waves are a dynamic exercise that targets the shoulders, arms, and core muscles, while also providing cardiovascular benefits.

How to Perform Battle Rope Waves:

- Stand with your feet hip-width apart and hold a battle rope in each hand, palms facing each other.
- Lower into a quarter-squat position with your knees slightly bent and your core engaged.
- Begin making waves with the ropes by moving your arms up and down in an alternating fashion.
- Continue for a set duration or number of repetitions, maintaining a steady rhythm.
- Aim for 20-30 seconds of continuous waves.

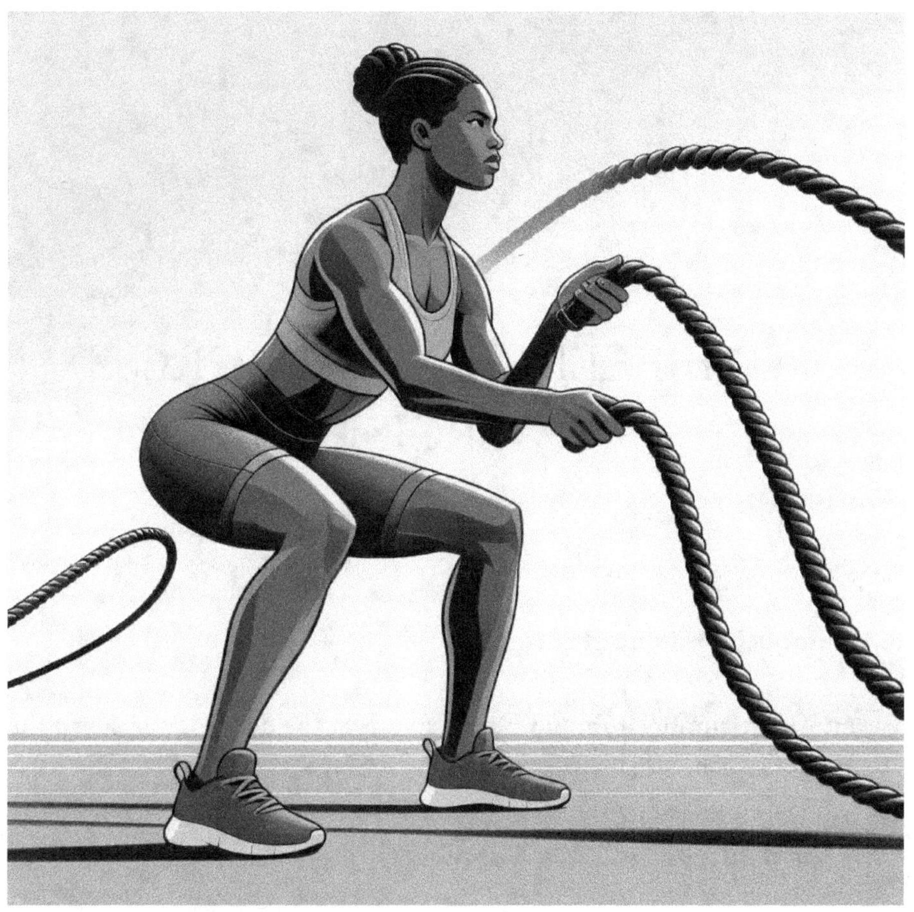

Benefits of Battle Rope Waves:

1. Strengthens shoulder and arm muscles.
2. Engages core muscles for stabilization.
3. Increases heart rate for cardiovascular benefits.

53

DUMBBELL SHOULDER PRESS EXERCISE

52) Dumbbell Shoulder Press:

Description: Dumbbell shoulder presses target the deltoid muscles of the shoulders, as well as the triceps and upper chest.

How to Perform of Dumbbell Shoulder Press:

- Sit or stand with your feet shoulder-width apart and hold a dumbbell in each hand at shoulder height.
- Press the dumbbells overhead until your arms are fully extended, but not locked out.
- Lower the dumbbells back down to shoulder height with control.
- Aim for 10-12 repetitions.

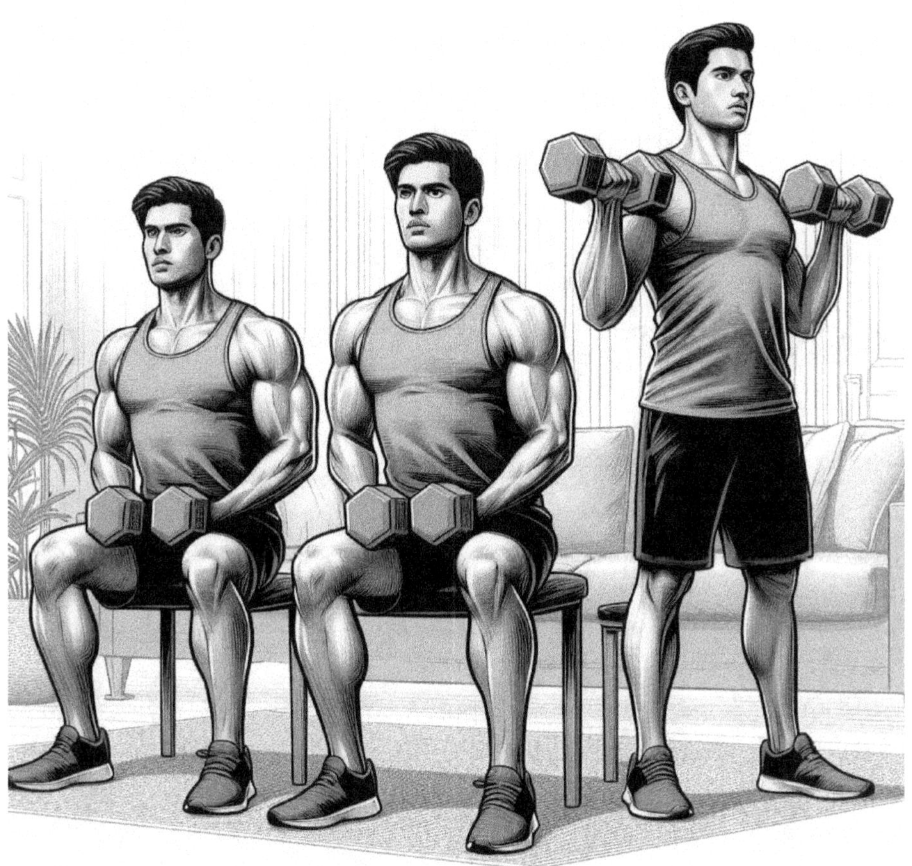

Benefits of Dumbbell Shoulder Press:

1. Strengthens shoulder muscles.
2. Improves upper body pressing strength.
3. Engages core muscles for stabilization.

54

RENEGADE ROWS WITH PUSH-UPS EXERCISE

53) Renegade Rows with Push-Ups:

Description: Renegade rows with push-ups combine the rowing motion of renegade rows with the pushing motion of push-ups, targeting the back, shoulders, arms, chest, and core muscles.

How to Perform Renegade Rows with Push-Ups:

- Start in a high plank position with a dumbbell in each hand, wrists aligned under shoulders.
- Perform one renegade row by rowing one dumbbell up towards your hip, retracting your shoulder blade.
- Lower the dumbbell back to the ground and perform one push-up.
- Continue alternating rows and push-ups while maintaining proper plank form.
- Aim for 8-10 repetitions on each side.

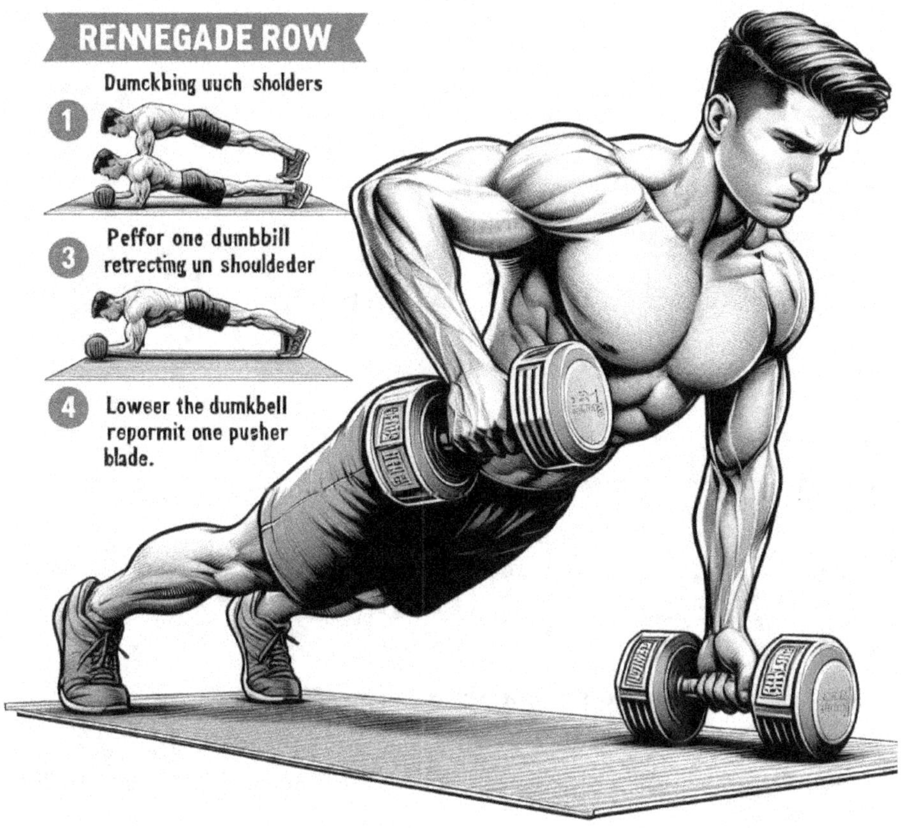

Benefits of Renegade Rows with Push-Ups:

1. Strengthens upper body muscles.
2. Engages core muscles for stabilization.
3. Challenges the cardiovascular system.

55

MEDICINE BALL SLAMS EXERCISE

54) Medicine Ball Slams:

Description: Medicine ball slams are a dynamic exercise that targets the entire body, including the core, shoulders, arms, and legs.

How to Perform Medicine Ball Slams:

- Stand with your feet hip-width apart and hold a medicine ball with both hands overhead.
- Explosively slam the medicine ball down towards the ground in front of you, using your core and upper body strength.
- Catch the ball on the bounce and immediately lift it back overhead to begin the next repetition.
- Aim for 12-15 repetitions.

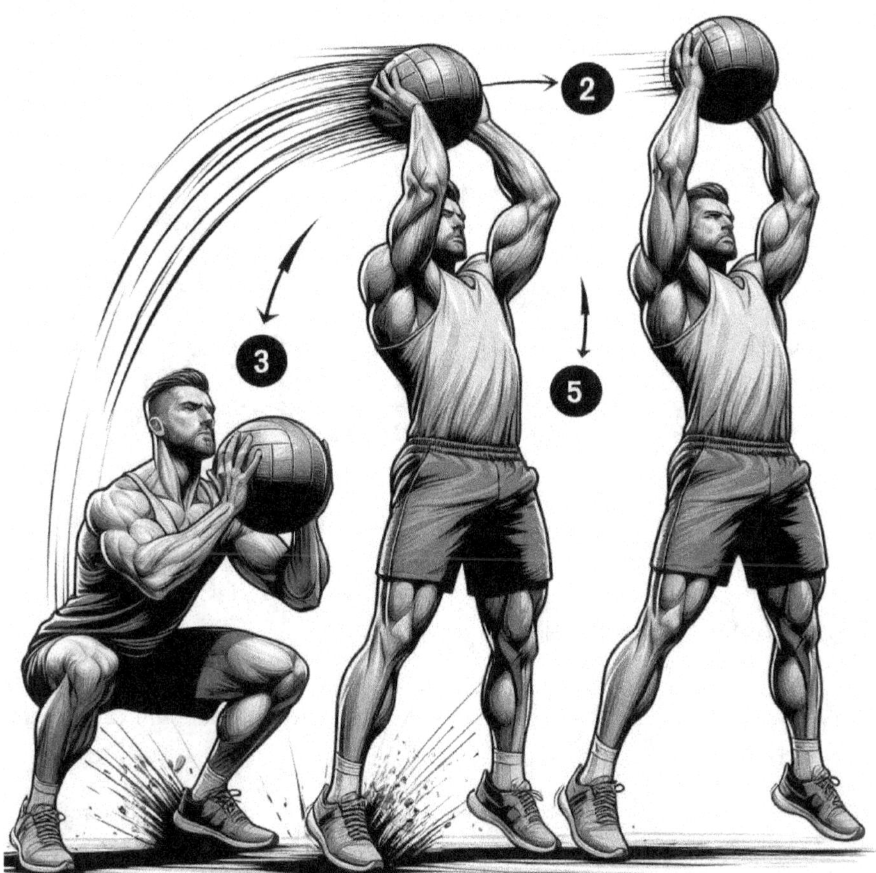

Benefits of Medicine Ball Slams:

1. Strengthens core muscles.
2. Improves upper body power and explosiveness.
3. Provides cardiovascular benefits.

56

SQUAT TO OVERHEAD PRESS EXERCISE

55) Squat to Overhead Press:

Description: Squat to overhead press is a compound exercise that targets the lower body, shoulders, and arms.

How to Perform Squat to Overhead Press:

- Hold a dumbbell or kettlebell in each hand at shoulder height, palms facing forward.
- Lower into a squat by bending your knees and sitting back into your hips.
- Push through your heels to return to standing, simultaneously pressing the weights overhead until your arms are fully extended.
- Lower the weights back to shoulder height and immediately lower into another squat to begin the next repetition.
- Aim for 10-12 repetitions.

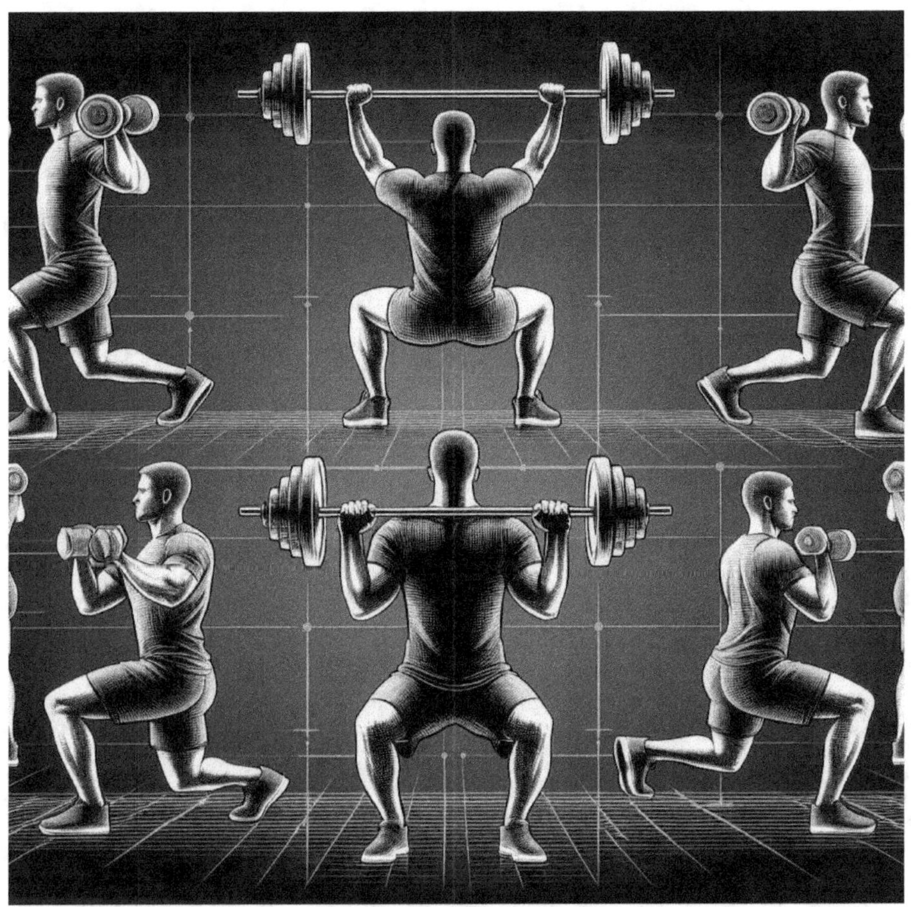

Benefits of Squat to Overhead Press:

1. Strengthens lower body muscles.
2. Improves upper body pressing strength.
3. Engages core muscles for stabilization.

57

SINGLE-LEG SQUATS (PISTOL SQUATS) WITH TRX EXERCISE

56) Single-Leg Squats (Pistol Squats) with TRX:

Description: Single-leg squats with TRX suspension straps are a challenging variation of the pistol squat that targets the quadriceps, hamstrings, glutes, and core muscles, while also improving balance and stability.

How to Perform Single-Leg Squats (Pistol Squats) with TRX:

- Hold onto the TRX handles with both hands and extend your arms straight out in front of you.
- Lift one foot off the ground and extend it straight out in front of you.
- Lower into a squat on the opposite leg, keeping your chest up and your back straight.
- Push through your heel to return to the starting position.
- Aim for 5-8 repetitions on each leg.

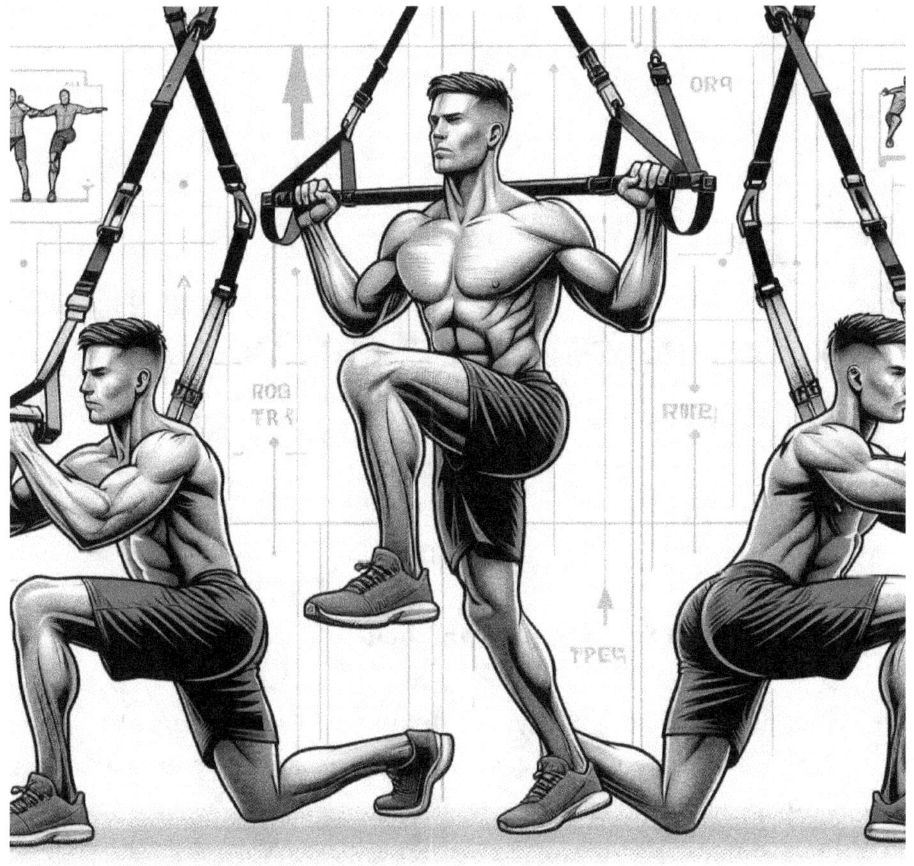

Benefits of Single-Leg Squats (Pistol Squats) with TRX:

1. Strengthens lower body muscles.
2. Improves balance and stability.
3. Challenges core muscles.

58

BULGARIAN SPLIT SQUATS WITH DUMBBELLS EXERCISE

57) Bulgarian Split Squats with Dumbbells:

Description: Bulgarian split squats with dumbbells are a unilateral lower body exercise that targets the quadriceps, hamstrings, glutes, and calves, while also improving balance and stability.

How to Perform Bulgarian Split Squats with Dumbbells:

- Stand facing away from a bench or elevated platform with a dumbbell in each hand.
- Place the top of one foot on the bench behind you, laces down.
- Lower into a lunge position on the opposite leg, bending both knees to approximately 90-degree angles.
- Push through your front heel to return to the starting position.
- Aim for 8-10 repetitions on each leg.

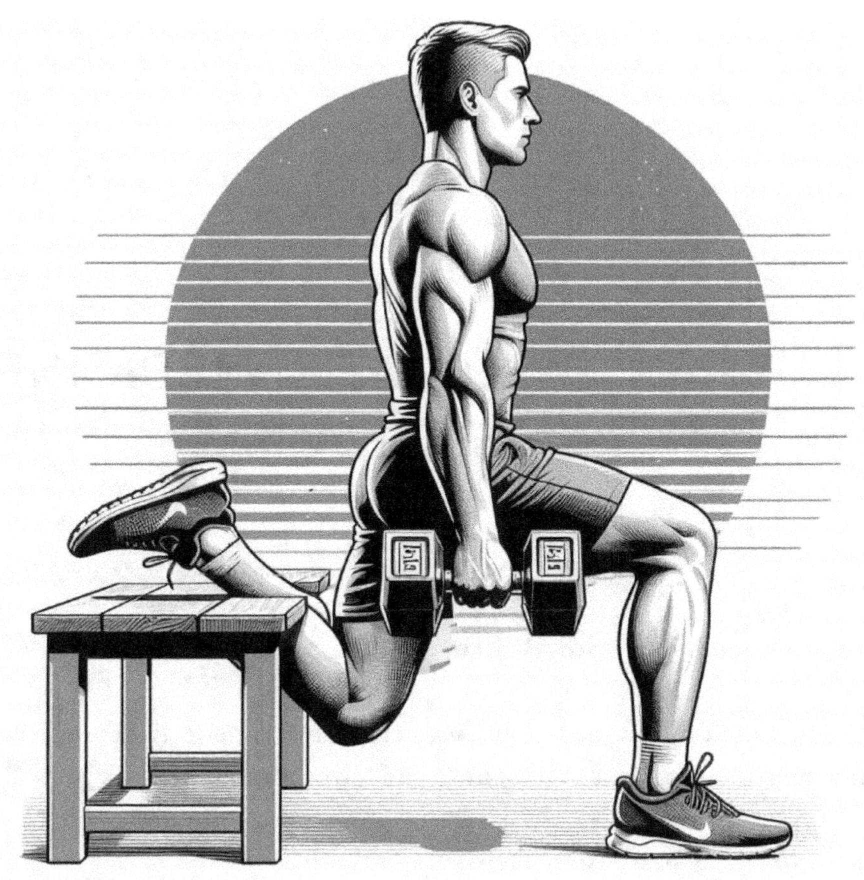

Benefits of Bulgarian Split Squats with Dumbbells:

1. Strengthens lower body muscles.
2. Improves balance and stability.
3. Corrects muscle imbalances between the left and right legs.

59

RUSSIAN TWISTS WITH MEDICINE BALLS EXERCISE

58) Russian Twists with Medicine Ball:

Description: Russian twists with a medicine ball are an effective core exercise that targets the obliques, abdominal, and lower back.

How to Perform Russian Twists with Medicine Ball:

- Sit on the ground with your knees bent and your feet flat on the floor, holding a medicine ball with both hands.
- Lean back slightly and lift your feet off the ground, balancing on your sit bones.
- Twist your torso to the right, bringing the medicine ball towards the ground beside your hip.
- Return to the center and twist to the left, bringing the medicine ball towards the ground beside your left hip.
- Continue alternating twists for the desired number of repetitions.

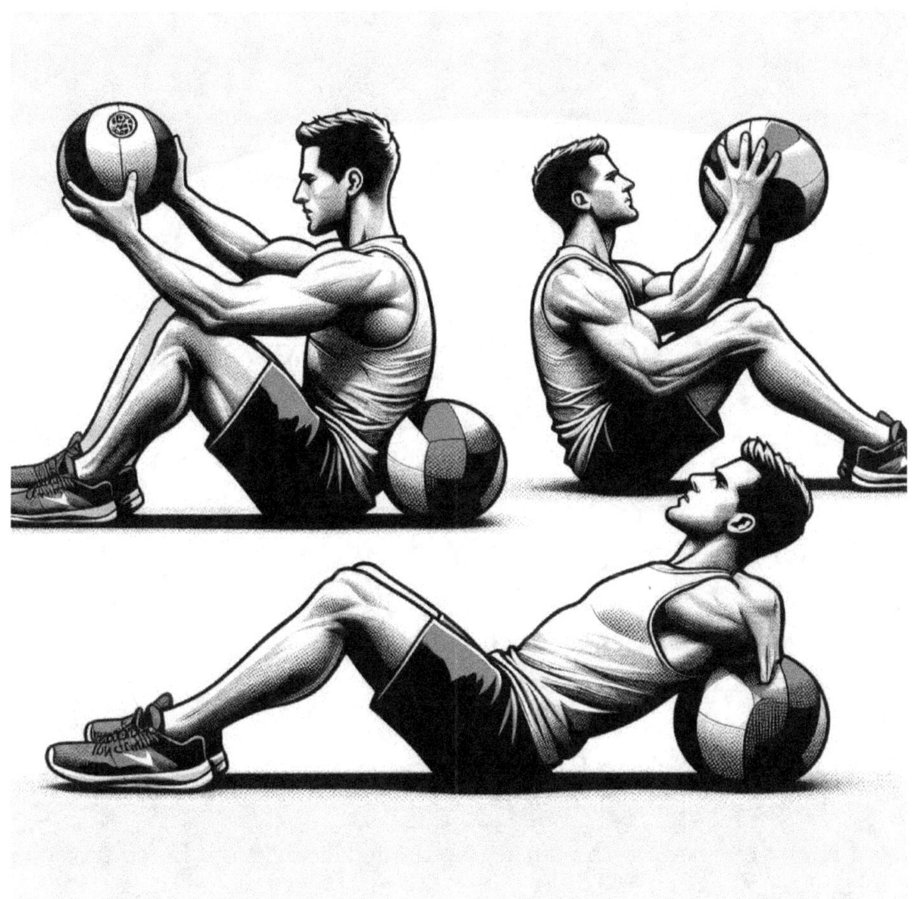

Benefits of Russian Twists with Medicine Ball:

1. Strengthens oblique muscles.
2. Improves rotational core strength.
3. Stabilizes the spine and improves posture.

60

SCISSOR KICKS EXERCISE

59) Scissor Kicks:

Description: Scissor kicks are a challenging core exercise that targets the lower abdominal and hip flexors.

How to Perform Scissor Kicks:

- Lie on your back with your legs extended straight out in front of you and your arms by your sides.
- Lift your legs a few inches off the ground and scissor them back and forth in an alternating fashion.
- Keep your lower back pressed into the floor throughout the movement and engage your core to stabilize your pelvis.
- Aim for 20-30 seconds of continuous movement.

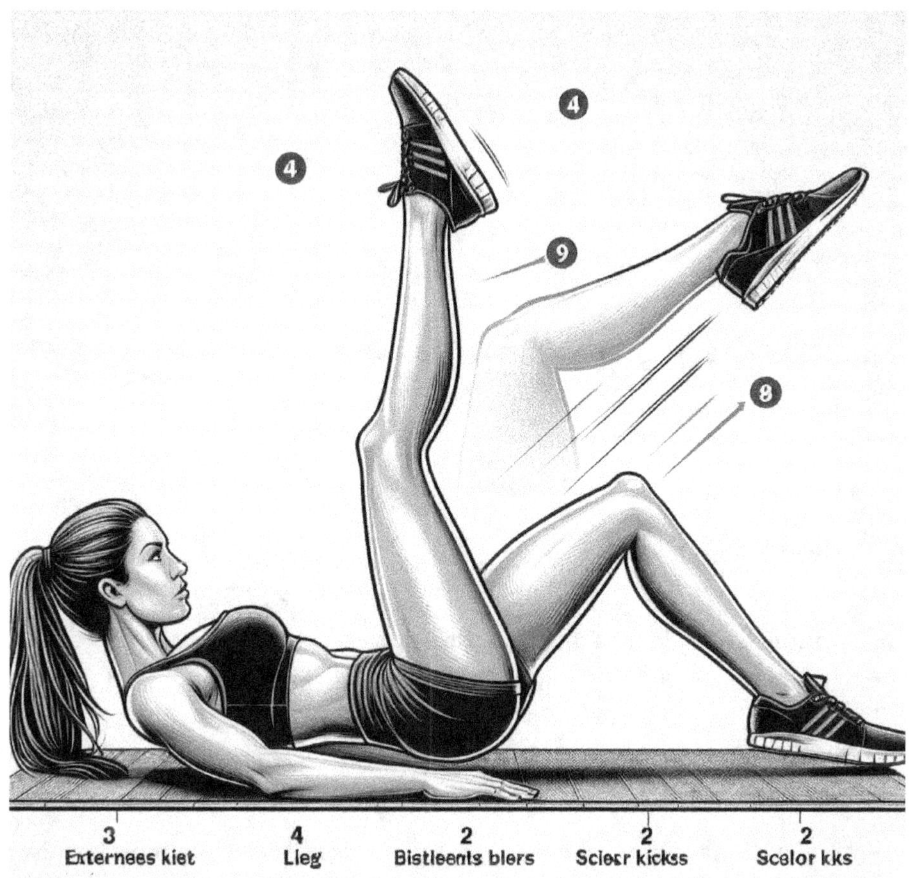

Benefits of Scissor Kicks:

1. Strengthens lower abdominal muscles.
2. Improves hip flexor strength and flexibility.
3. Stabilizes the pelvis and lower back.

61

TRICEPS KICKBACKS EXERCISE

60) Tricep Kickbacks:

Description: Tricep kickbacks are an isolation exercise that targets the triceps, helping to tone and strengthen the back of the arms.

How to Perform Tricep Kickbacks:

- Hold a dumbbell in each hand and hinge forward at the hips, keeping your back flat and your chest up.
- Bend your elbows to bring the dumbbells towards your sides, then extend your arms straight back behind you, squeezing your triceps at the top of the movement.
- Lower the dumbbells back down with control and repeat for the desired number of repetitions.
- Aim for 10-12 repetitions.

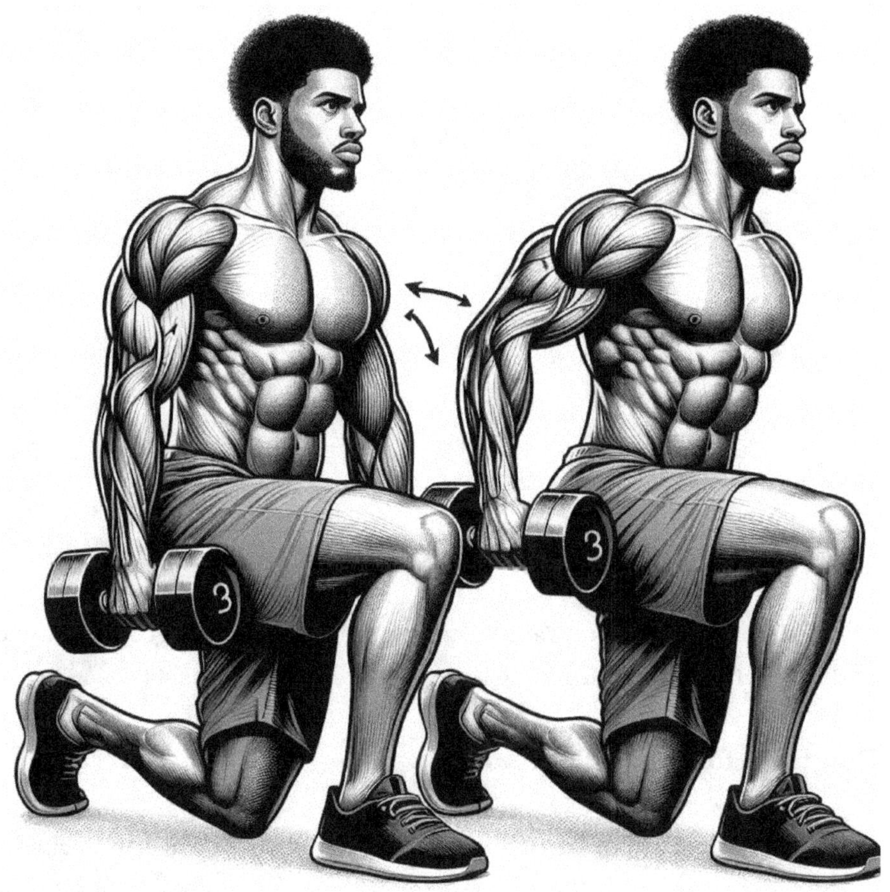

Benefits of Tricep Kickbacks:

1. Targets and tones triceps muscles.
2. Helps improve arm definition and strength.
3. Can be performed with minimal equipment.

62

BENT OVER ROWS EXERCISE

61) Bent Over Rows:

Description: Bent over rows are a compound exercise that targets the muscles of the upper back, including the lats, rhomboids, and traps.

How to Perform Bent Over Rows:

- Hold a dumbbell or barbell in front of you with an overhand grip and hinge forward at the hips, keeping your back flat and your chest up.
- Bend your elbows and pull the weight towards your lower rib cage, squeezing your shoulder blades together at the top of the movement.
- Lower the weight back down with control and repeat for the desired number of repetitions.
- Aim for 10-12 repetitions.

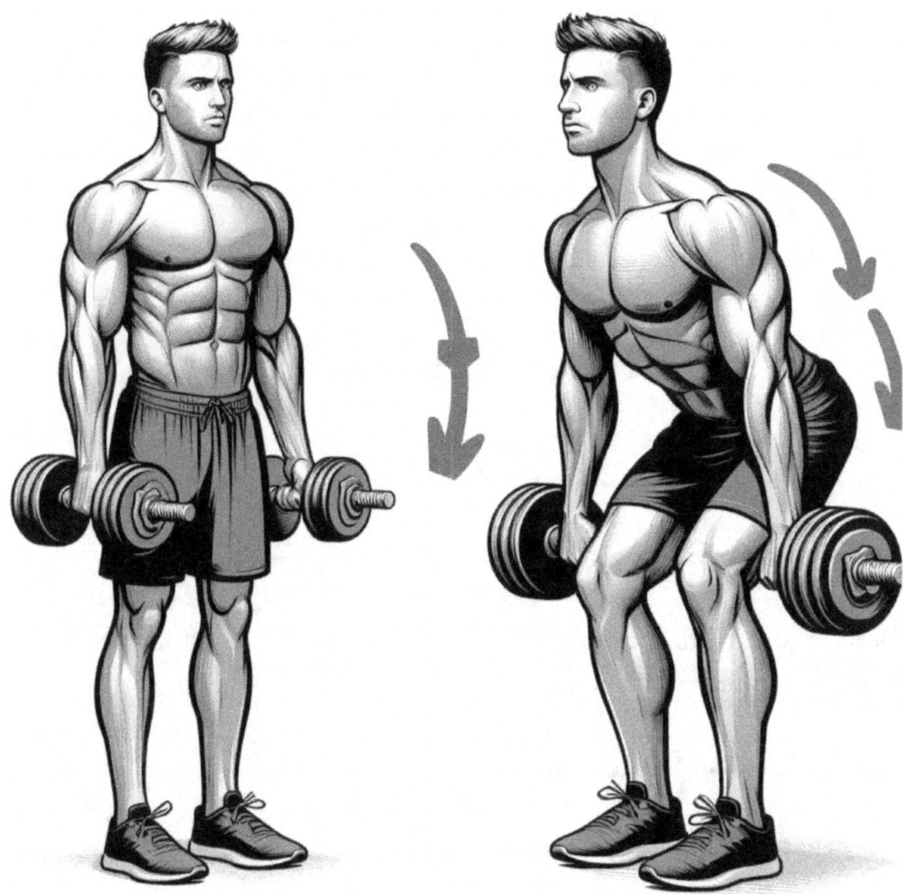

Benefits of Bent Over Rows:

1. Strengthens upper back muscles.
2. Improves posture and spinal alignment.
3. Engages core muscles for stabilization.

63

FLUTTER KICKS EXERCISE

62) Flutter Kicks:

Description: Flutter kicks are a challenging core exercise that targets the lower abdominals and hip flexors.

How to Perform Flutter Kicks:

- Lie on your back with your legs extended straight out in front of you and your arms by your sides.
- Lift your legs a few inches off the ground and flutter them up and down in an alternating fashion.
- Keep your lower back pressed into the floor throughout the movement and engage your core to stabilize your pelvis.
- Aim for 20-30 seconds of continuous movement.

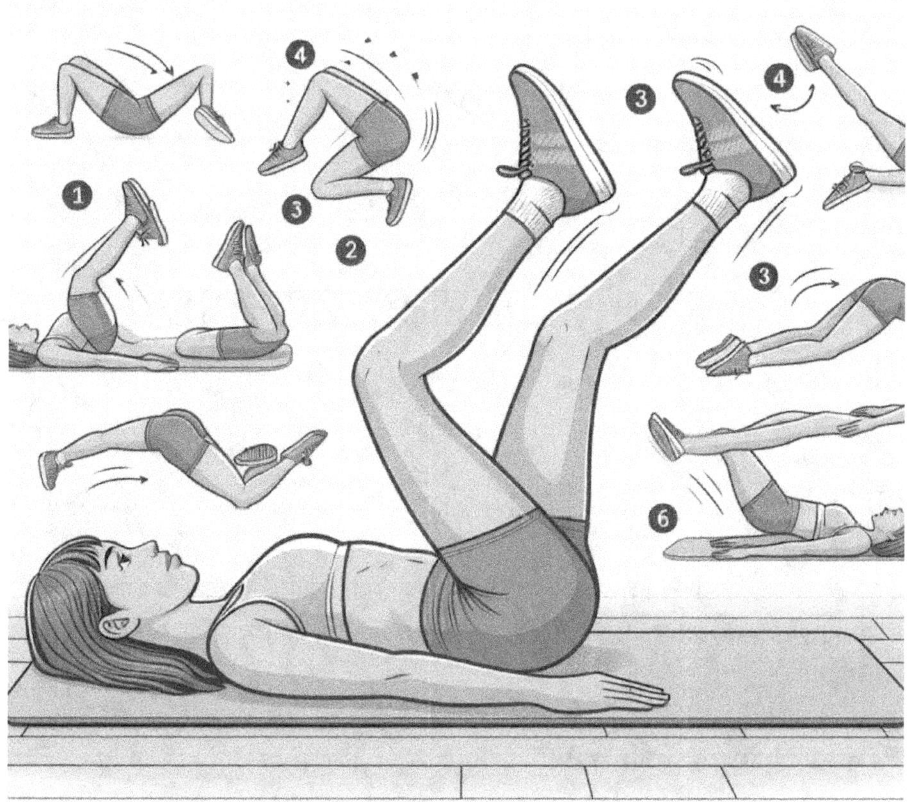

Benefits of Flutter Kicks:

1. Strengthens lower abdominal muscles.
2. Improves hip flexor strength and flexibility.
3. Stabilizes the pelvis and lower back.

64

CRAB WALKS EXERCISE

63) Crab Walks:

Description: Crab walks are a full-body exercise that targets the muscles of the upper body, core, and lower body, while also improving coordination and agility.

How to Perform Crab Walks:

- Sit on the ground with your knees bent and your feet flat on the floor, placing your hands behind you with your fingers pointing towards your body.
- Lift your hips off the ground and walk forward by moving your hands and feet in an alternating fashion, maintaining a stable core throughout.
- Continue walking forward for a set distance or time, then reverse direction and walk backward.
- Aim for 20-30 seconds of crab walks.

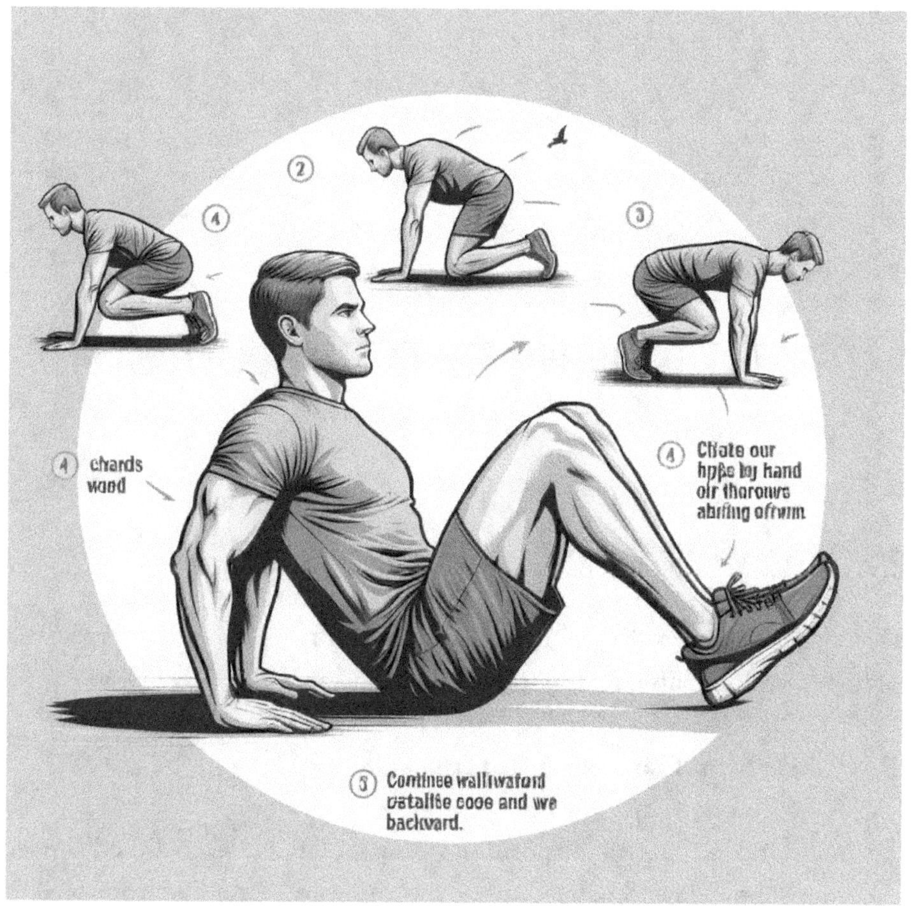

Benefits of Crab Walks:

1. Strengthens upper body muscles.
2. Engages core muscles for stabilization.
3. Improves coordination and agility.

65

PLANK WITH HIP DIPS EXERCISE

64) Plank with Hip Dips:

Description: Plank with hip dips is a dynamic core exercise that targets the obliques, abdominals, and hip stabilizers.

How to Perform Plank with Hip Dips:

- You stand in a high plank position with your hands placed directly under your shoulders and with your body forming a straight line from head to heels.
- Engage your core and rotate your hips to one side, lowering them towards the ground without letting them touch.
- Return to the starting position, then rotate your hips to the other side and lower towards the ground.
- Continue alternating hip dips while maintaining proper plank form.
- Aim for 10-12 dips on each side.

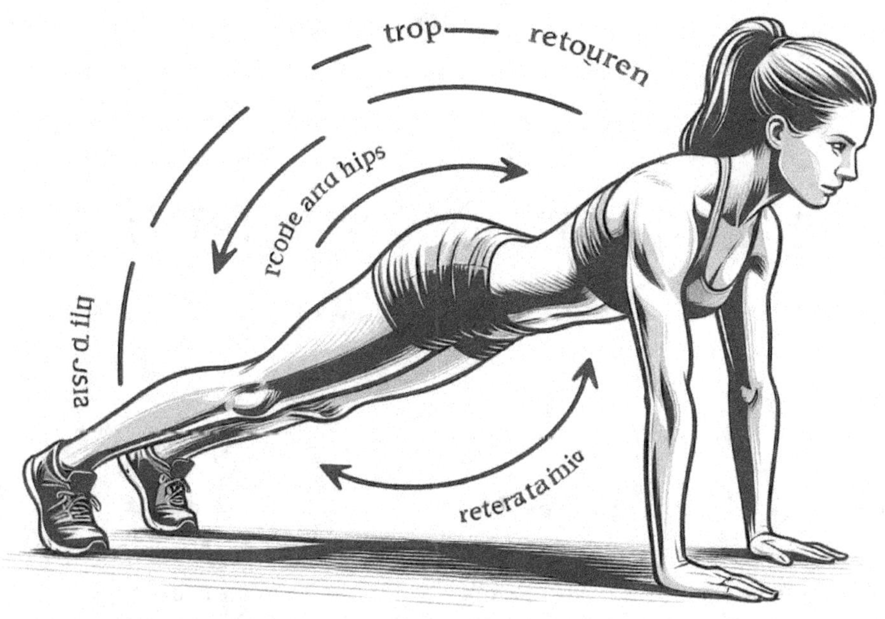

Benefits of Plank with Hip Dips:

1. Strengthens oblique muscles.
2. Improves core stability and strength.
3. Engages hip stabilizers for balance.

66

PLANK WITH REACH THROUGH EXERCISE

65) Plank with Reach Through:

Description: The Plank with Reach Through is a dynamic exercise focused on strengthening your core, targeting the abdominals, obliques, shoulders, and arms.

How to Perform Plank with Reach Through:

- Commence in a high plank position, ensuring your hands are directly beneath your shoulders, and your body forms a straight line from head to heels.
- Activate your core muscles and elevate one arm from the ground, extending it beneath your body and across to the opposite side.
- Return to the initial position, then repeat the movement with the opposite arm, extending it beneath your body and across to the other side.
- Continue alternating reach-throughs while maintaining proper plank form.
- Aim for 10-12 repetitions on each side.

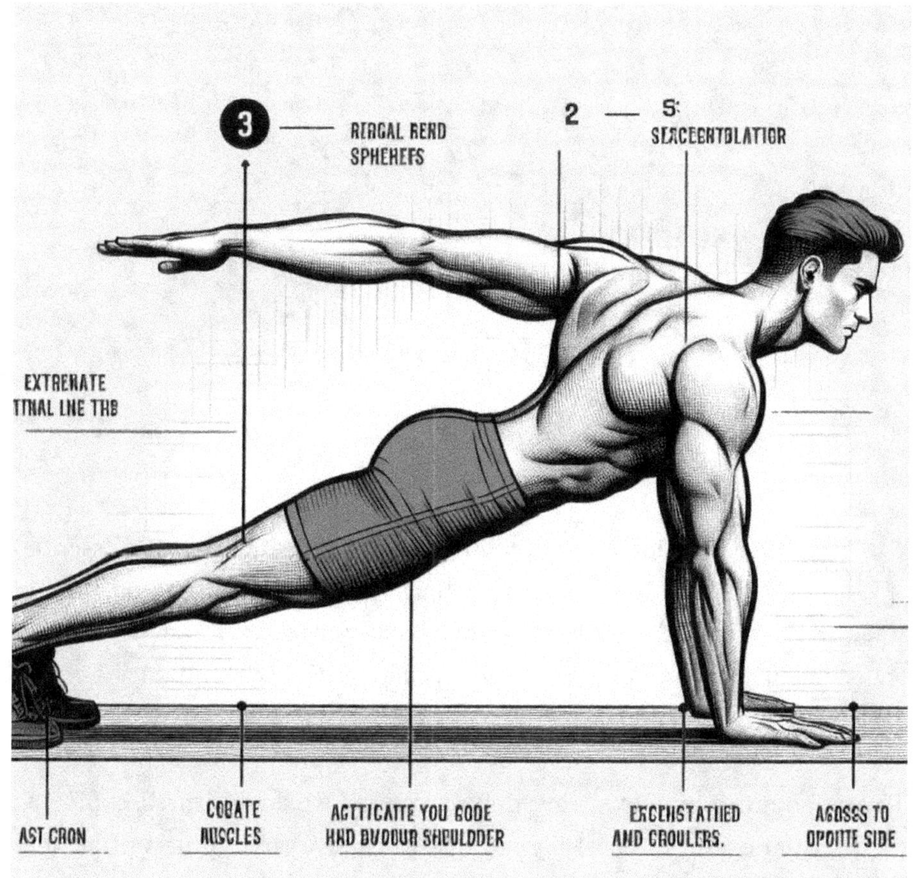

Benefits of Plank with Reach Through:

1. Enhances core muscle strength.
2. Involves shoulder and arm muscles for stabilization.
3. Improves shoulder mobility and flexibility.

67

CONCLUSION

Congratulations on reaching the conclusion of "65 Essential Simple Exercises for Every Stage of Life - Strength and Vitality Assured"! As we wrap up this journey together, let's reflect on the transformative power of exercise and the incredible potential it holds for each and every one of us.

Throughout this book, we have delved into the world of fitness, exploring 65 essential exercises carefully curated to cater to individuals of all ages and fitness levels. From young adults seeking to build a solid foundation of strength and vitality to seniors striving to maintain their mobility and independence, these exercises offer a gateway to a healthier, happier life at every stage.

As we have learned, the benefits of regular exercise extend far beyond mere physical fitness. Yes, these exercises are designed to strengthen our muscles, improve our flexibility, and boost our cardiovascular health. But they also hold the power to uplift our spirits, sharpen our minds, and invigorate our souls.

Consider the simple act of starting your day with a few minutes of stretching or engaging in a brisk walk around the neighborhood. These seemingly small gestures have the potential to set the tone for the entire day, infusing us with energy, clarity, and a sense of purpose that carries us through even the most challenging moments.

But perhaps the most profound lesson we have learned is that exercise is not just something we do; it's a way of life. It's about showing up for ourselves each and every day, honoring our bodies, and nurturing our well-being in mind, body, and spirit.

As you reflect on the exercises you have encountered in this book, I encourage you to see them not as mere physical movements but as opportunities for growth, transformation, and self-discovery. Embrace each exercise with an open heart and a curious mind, allowing yourself to fully experience the joy, the challenge, and the exhilaration that comes with moving your body and embracing your strength.

And remember, the journey to strength and vitality is not always easy. There might be days when you feel tired, discouraged, or even tempted to give up. However, it's during those challenging moments that your authentic resilience becomes evident. It's when you dig deep, push past your limits, and keep moving forward that you discover just how resilient and capable you truly are.

So, as we bid farewell to "65 Essential Simple Exercises for Every Stage of Life - Strength and Vitality Assured," let us carry with us the knowledge, the wisdom, and the inspiration gleaned from these pages. Let us commit to making exercise a priority in our lives, knowing that each step we take, each rep we complete, brings us one step closer to the vibrant, vital life we deserve.

I want to sincerely thank you for embarking on this journey with me. May your path be filled with strength, vitality, and boundless joy, today and always.

68

REFERENCES

1. Forbes Health. (2023). 4 Exercises To Try While Traveling. [online] Available at: https://www.forbes.com/health/fitness/travel-friendly-exercise-ideas.

2. How To Unlock Your Push Up Strength (In 5 Minutes) | BOXROX. (n.d.). Www.boxrox.com. Retrieved February 5, 2024, from https://www.boxrox.com/how-to-unlock-your-push-up-strength-in-5-minutes

3. Plank Exercises for Fitness - Health and Fitness Today. (2023, May 19). Healthandfitness.today. https://healthandfitness.today/plank-exercises-for-fitness

4. Kinesiology of the Seated Row Exercise. (n.d.). KinX Learning. Retrieved February 5, 2024, from https://kinxlearning.com/pages/seated-row

5. 21 At-Home Arm Exercises: With and Without Weights. (2020, November 23). Greatist. https://greatist.com/fitness/exercises-at-home-for-arms

6. How At-Home Calisthenics Can Take Your Sports Performance to the Next Level. (n.d.). Www.topendsports.com. Retrieved February 5, 2024, from https://www.topendsports.com/fitness/calisthenics.htm

7. Manchanda, Y. (2023, May 7). Benefits of up downs: Strengthen your entire body with this exercise. Www.sportskeeda.com. https://www.sp

ortskeeda.com/health-and-fitness/benefits-downs-strengthen-entire-body-exercise

8. Dabus, Z. (2023, December 22). 10 Effective Gym Exercises for Strengthening Your Core. Max Fitness Auburn, AL. https://www.maxfitnessauburn.com/10-effective-gym-exercises-for-strengthening-your-core

9. 5 Highly Effective Oblique Exercises Better than Crunches | BOXROX. (n.d.). Www.boxrox.com. Retrieved February 5, 2024, from https://www.boxrox.com/5-super-effective-oblique-exercises-better-than-crunches

10. updated, S. H. last. (2023, September 23). This abs workout for beginners sculpts a strong core in 4 moves and 20 minutes. Tom's Guide. https://www.tomsguide.com/features/this-4-move-abs-workout-for-beginners-strengthens-your-core-in-20-minutes

11. What are the most effective tummy twister exercises for reducing belly fat? (2019). Quora. https://www.quora.com/What-are-the-most-effective-tummy-twister-exercises-for-reducing-belly-fat

12. 24 Ab Workouts At Home Without Equipment Needed| Online Class. (2023, August 12). https://fitwithursula.com/24-ab-workouts-at-home-no-equipment-needed

13. Bench Dips. (n.d.). Totalworkout.fitness. Retrieved February 5, 2024, from https://totalworkout.fitness/en/exercise/10661

14. Claxton, J. (2022, October 3). Wall Push-Ups: How To, Benefits, Variations & Muscles Worked. https://fitnessdy.com/wall-push-ups

15. Strengthen Your Lower Back: 20 Engaging Exercises to Strengthen Lower Back. (2023, July 12). Mainstay Medical. https://mainstaymedical.com/exercises-to-strengthen-lower-back